*This book is dedicated
to our families*

Springer
Milano
Berlin
Heidelberg
New York
Barcelona
Budapest
Hong Kong
London
Paris
Santa Clara
Singapore
Tokyo

Francesco Capasso • Timothy S. Gaginella

Laxatives
A Practical Guide

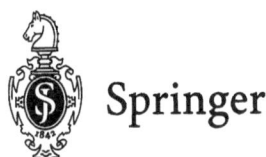 Springer

FRANCESCO CAPASSO
Department of Experimental
Pharmacology
University of Naples "Federico II"
Naples, Italy

TIMOTHY S. GAGINELLA
School of Pharmacy
University of Wisconsin
Madison, Wisconsin
USA

ISBN-13: 978-3-540-75037-6   e-ISBN-13: 978-88-470-2227-0
DOI: 10.1007/978-88-470-2227-0

Library of Congress Cataloging-in-Publication Data. Capasso, Francesco. Laxatives: a prati-
cal guide/Francesco Capasso, Timothy S. Gaginella. p. cm. Includes bibliographical references and index. 1. Laxatives. I. Gaginella, Timothy S. II. Title.
[DNLM: 1. Cathartics--pharmacology. 2. Cathartics--therapeutic use. 3. Constipation--drug therapy. QV 75 C236L 1997] RM357.C36 1997 615'.732--dc21 DNLM/DLC for Library of
Congress 97-3681 CIP

© Springer-Verlag Italia, Milano 1997

Preface

Constipation is a common disorder that is often defined differently by patients and physicians. Clinically, constipation occurs when bowel movements are difficult or painful. The "normality" of bowel movements, in terms of frequency, varies among individuals; frequency that is thought by one person to be *constipation* may be reported by another to be usual and thus normal. Often the perceived "need" to have a bowel movement leads to self-treatment with laxatives as these drugs are widely available without a prescription. This situation can raise problems in patient care, because of potential interactions between laxatives and other medications. Furthermore, chronic use (abuse) of laxatives can cause serious medical consequences, causing patients to visit physicians, and even to be hospitalized for further evaluation and care. This has a financial impact on the patient, and on health care systems. It is essential that pharmacists, physicians and other health care practitioners counsel patients on the causes of constipation and the proper use of laxatives. A medical work-up by a physician should be done to determine if the constipation is due to a pathological process. Often normal bowel function (for an invididual) can be maintained by diet and/or lifestyle.

Most laxatives in use today are of botanical origin. Further research on the mechanism of action of these and synthetic laxatives is needed to better define their pharmacology and toxicology. While research continues, we trust that this book will serve medical professionals as a practical guide to laxatives and their proper use in treating constipation. It is our hope that judicious use of laxatives will not only benefit patients but will also reduce the cost of delivering health care.

We express our appreciation to Springer-Verlag for the helpful suggestions and enthusiasm which made this monograph possible.

Francesco Capasso
Timothy S. Gaginella

Contents

1. Introduction

Millions of persons worldwide suffer from difficult or painful defecation, known commonly as constipation. Although the frequency of bowel movements varies greatly among normal healthy individuals, it is usual for those with constipation to voluntarily (because of physical discomfort) or involuntarily (because of disease, drugs or the stress of daily life) delay defecation. The absence of enough fiber in the diet, the lack of physical exercise and insufficient fluid intake also contribute to constipation.

Laxatives are drugs that treat constipation through facilitation of defecation. Even though there is a real medical need for treating constipation and for preparing the bowel for endoscopic examination, laxatives are commonly used inappropriately. The general public, often overly concerned about maintaining a daily bowel movement, lacks the proper education to evaluate when a real need exists for the use of a laxative. Particularly the elderly tend to self-prescribe laxatives, contributing to these drugs being the most widely used of all nonprescription products. The availability of a diversity of nonprescription laxative preparations adds to the popularity of these drugs. In 1973 only 130 million dollars were spent on laxatives in the United States, 492 million dollars (Moriarty and Silk, 1988) were spent in 1985 and in 1996 this amount was already more than 500 million dollars. In 1995 about 1120 million lire were spent for laxatives in Italy. In Germany 49 million German marks were spent on senna products in 1990, representing 40% of the entire laxative market (Leng-Peschlow 1992). It has been estimated that in Great Britain about 25% of the healthy population use laxatives. On the other hand every year about 4% of the adult population visit a physician or a pharmacist because of constipation. This rate increases to 8% in the elderly, with women attending twice as frequently as men. Although most constipation is not associated with defined illness, these figures emphasize the importance of laxatives in Western society and the need for patients, pharmacists, nurses and physicians to be better informed about the pharmacognosy and pharmacology of these important drugs.

To the casual reader it might appear that a discussion of constipation and laxatives would be rather straightforward and unencumbered by complex medical or scientific explanations. This apparent simplicity in dealing with the subject of bowel movements is deceptive. This is principally because of antiquated definitions and overly naive explanations for how material moves through the gastrointestinal tract.

1.1 Definitions

Most readers probably feel confident that they could easily define *absorption*, *secretion* and *motility*. The term "motility" is particularly confusing. Logically, an increase in motility should increase movement of the intestine but the term does not define the direction or nature of the movement. Thus, an increase in motility of the small intestine can be nonpropulsive (causing no movement of intraluminal material in the direction of the rectum). Increased motility of the circular muscle can actually obstruct the lumen and produce an effect opposite to what might be anticipated. It is the transit of material through the lumen that is most important. This is controlled by the coordinated activity of the various smooth muscle components of the intestine.

What is absorption? Is it merely the movement of a substance from the lumen into the epithelial cells or does it refer to transfer of a substance from the lumen into the blood? What about secretion? This occurs throughout the gastrointestinal tract under normal circumstances, but is it decreased in constipation and increased in response to laxatives or in diarrhea? Which portion of the intestinal tract is most important in determining whether a change in absorption or secretion will result in constipation or diarrhea? Whether the intestinal mucosa is absorbing or secreting will define the fluidity of the intestinal contents. While the terms absorption/secretion and motility are important, assessment of constipation and laxation is most accurate when based upon the amount of fluid in the luminal contents and the rate of transit through the intestinal tract.

1.2 Laxative classification: Is it necessary?

Over the years attempts to classify laxatives have created more confusion than clarity. The most traditional classification has placed substances in the categories of *bulk-forming agents, osmotic laxatives, stimulants/irritants* and *lubricants*. In the last 25 years we have gained sufficient knowledge about the mechanisms of action of laxatives to know that most of these drugs have multiple effects that result in laxation. Therefore, it is difficult, if not impossible, to use this simplistic classification.

Laxatives increase the fluid content of the bowel and most also directly or indirectly (due to fluid accumulation) alter motility (Gaginella 1995a). Therefore, it is not appropriate to merely categorize laxatives as motility-enhancing agents or intestinal secretagogues, at least not in a mutually exclusive sense. Use of the terms "irritant" and "stimulant" is inappropriate (Gaginella and Bass 1978; Leng-Peschlow 1992) because there is little scientific basis for defining the tissues and cells that are the object of the stimulation and "irritation". On the other hand, *stimulation* is inherent to every pharmacological action. In this sense all laxatives can be considered stimulants, whether they stimulate the bowel by physical forces (bulking agents), by osmotic action (osmotically active, poorly absorbable molecules) or by chemical effects (castor oil, anthranoids, diphenylmethanes). Accordingly, it is incorrect to classify together drugs such as castor oil and the diphenylmethanes, which cause mucosal lesions (e.g. epithelial cell loss), with drugs such as the anthraquinones, for which there is little evidence of tissue injury. Likewise, "irritant" could just as well be used to describe the action of hypertonic saline solutions, as could "osmotic" laxative.

Several options for grouping laxative drugs exist. They may be grouped as to **chemical class** (sugars and sugar alcohols, nonabsorbable polysaccharides, bile acids, hydroxylated fatty acids, inorganic salts, molecules with anthranoid structure, derivatives of diphenylmethane), **site of action** (small intestine, large intestine, whole intestinal tract), **mode of action** (bulk forming agents, lubricants, osmotics, stimulants/irritants), **intensity of effect** (laxative, cathartic, purgative) or **origin** (natural, synthetic). The first grouping, chemical class, does not take into account drugs such as natural fibers or fruits and other foods that contain a mixture of active components. The site of action of a laxative could be an important criterion, because constipation is mainly a large bowel problem and laxatives should therefore act predominantly on the large bowel. However, the site of action grouping is not useful because most laxatives act in more than one portion of the bowel and they may have an effect on fluid secretion in one area and alter motility in another. If the drug works throughout the bowel then one does not need classification based on site of action. "Mode of action" sounds like an attractive way to group these drugs but the argument above illustrates the error in using terms like stimulant; most of these drugs work by **multiple** modes of action.

"Intensity of effect" is not a reasonable term either. The ancient literature up to the eighteenth century includes references to *drastics, cathartics, aperients* and *purgatives* in addition to laxatives. Texts in the twentieth century are more apt to have deleted the terms drastics and aperients. The different terms were originally intended to indicate intensity, so that a mild effect on the bowels was produced by aperients or laxatives, and increasingly harsh effects were said to be produced by cathartics, purgatives and drastics (Travell 1954). These definitions merely confuse the understanding of how drugs bring about relief from constipation and they should be abandoned (Gaginella and Bass 1978). A singular term, *laxative*, should be used. Pharmacologically, laxatives can then be compared on a relative potency basis, because whether a laxative has a mild or harsh effect on the intestinal tract is related more to the dose administered than to major differences in intrinsic activity.

We believe it is best to discuss laxatives as to source, natural or synthetic (Table 1). The pharmacology of individual laxatives can then be discussed without the need to force a drug into a paradigm. Each can be freely described in terms of effects on the intestinal mucosa and muscle. The reader will

Table 1. Dosage and onset of action of natural and synthetic laxatives

Laxatives/Origin	Average adult dose (oral)	Onset of action (hours)
Natural laxatives		
Anthraquinones	250 mg	6 - 12
Castor oil	15-60 mL	2 - 6
Bran	20 g	12 - 72
Psyllium	4-30 g	12 - 72
Magnesium salts	2-30 g	0.5 - 3
Sodium phosphate	4-8 g	0.5 - 3
Mineral oil	15-45 mL	6 - 8
Synthetic laxatives		
Phenolphthalein	60-100 mg	6 - 8
Bisacodyl	30 mg	6 - 8
Danthron	75-150 mg	6 - 12
Dioctyl sulfosuccinate salts	50-500 mg	24 - 72
Sorbitol	20-50 g	24 - 48
Lactulose	15-60 mL	24 - 48
Methylcellulose	4-6 g	12 - 72
Polyethylene glycol	3 L	1

be able to easily identify whether the laxative is natural or synthetic and compare relative activities among laxatives of the anthraquinone, natural fiber, inorganic salt and other groups.

We have deliberately chosen not to exhaustingly reference every effect of the laxatives included in this monograph. Some general background is presented to form a framework for discussing the pharmacology of common (and some not so common) laxatives. Emphasis is on oral formulations. Although the bowel can be evacuated with suppositories or enemas, these methods are not treated in this volume.

2. Constipation: The Rationale for Laxative Use

It is not easy to define constipation; everyone seems to have their own concept based upon personal experience. The frequency of bowel movements varies greatly in individuals, so that "constipation" for one person may be normal for another. Some patients complain of an uneasy or a full feeling in the abdomen and believe they are constipated, even though they have had a bowel movement that day or the day before. Others may have a bowel movement every day but, because the stool is small in amount or requires straining to pass, they claim to be constipated. According to Thompson (1979) who studied the average frequency of bowel movements among the general population (post office employees, nurses, London factory workers and rural patients), about 70% had daily bowel movements, of which 7% considered themselves constipated, despite the fact few reported hard or infrequent stools. Twenty percent of the subjects in these groups used laxatives regularly. There is a rather antiquated idea, especially among many elderly patients, that it is healthy and necessary to have a bowel movement every day. This has contributed to confusion by preoccupying these individuals with unfounded concern that they need a laxative if they go more than a day without a bowel movement.

Constipation must be considered a symptom, not a disease process. It may mean (i) diminished frequency compared to what is considered normal, (ii) a smaller volume than what is considered normal, (iii) a lack of urgency to evacuate, (iv) difficulty with fecal expulsion, (v) a sense of incomplete evacuation, as well as (vi) multiple somatic complaints during days without defecation.

Attempts have been made to define constipation clinically in terms of stool weight, consistency, transit time and effort involved in having a bowel movement (Haubrich 1985). Stool weight and consistency are not good indicators. Likewise, effort in elimination is fraught with problems, mostly associated to the individual's perception of the degree of effort. What may be considered a difficult bowel movement for one individual may be considered quite normal for another. Clinically, transit time is a useful indicator of bowel function, the slowing down of which, in association with a reduced number of small volume stools, may aid in the diagnosis of constipation. However the time and expense associated with doing transit studies make such analyses impractical for the majority of patients complaining of this symptom.

The colon is commonly blamed for many ills. It is believed to be the controlling factor in causing constipation. In 1930 Campbell and Detwiller authored a book entitled *The Lazy Colon. Newer Methods and Latest Advances of Science in the Treatment of Constipation* which emphasized the need for frequent bowel movements to cleanse the body of toxins that would otherwise lead to illnesses from fatigue to high blood pressure. To prevent "autointoxication", it was suggested in the early part of this century that children two to three years of age have their large intestine and appendix surgically removed!

Is constipation a motility disorder, a disorder of altered absorptive/secretory functions of the colon , or a combination of both factors? Which portion(s) of the colon is (are) affected to bring about the constipation? We know that normally the basic tone, rhythmic segmentation and infrequent mass peristalsis move semi fluid material to the left colon while removing much of the water, so that the stool normally contains about 70% water and is easily passed. Based upon findings of changes in pressure within the colon, functional constipation has been categorized as "spastic" or "hypotonic", the former being the result of excessive segmental contraction of the lower colon and the latter due to reduced contractions and often associated with chronic use of laxatives (Thompson 1979). This type of constipation is common in irritable bowel syndrome. It is also present in children, businessmen and other travelers who, because of busy schedules without an appropriate time to visit the toilet, voluntarily delay defecation. Other causes for functional constipation are a lack of sufficient fluid intake, inactivity, pregnancy, depression, laxative abuse, low residue diet and age. In some cases it is due to a deficiency in generating sufficient abdominal pressure (Anderson 1986; Burgess 1972).

Organic causes of constipation are outlined in Table 2. In a general sense, the causes may be obstruction (e.g. carcinoma) or retention (e.g. proctitis or other physical or inflammatory conditions of the lower rectum or anus), or of metabolic (e.g. endocrine disorders), neurogenic or pharmacologic nature. Constipation is a common problem during pregnancy, mainly in the last 6 months (Parry et al. 1970; Wald et al. 1982; Lawson et al. 1985), and is ascribed to pressure from the uterus on the intestine, decreased intestinal muscle tone, lack of exercise and dietary changes (Burgess 1972). Constipation is often caused by drugs (iatrogenic constipation). The drugs that can cause constipation fall into a broad range of categories (Table 3). Opiate analgesics stimulate contraction of intestinal circular muscle, restricting the flow of luminal contents. Anticholinergics block the influence of acetylcholine on intestinal secretion and motility; tricyclic antidepressants also act through this mechanism. Diuretics act to dessicate the feces by increasing ion and water absorption or inhibiting secretion. Anti-Parkinson's disease drugs, antihypertensives, monoamine oxidase inhibitors, antipsychotics and ganglionic blockers act by altering the release or action of autonomic neurotransmitters on the intestinal mucosa and smooth muscle. Drugs like cholestyramine act to lower serum cholesterol by binding luminal bile acids; this prevents the bile acids from stimulating fluid secretion. Iron and bismuth produce

Table 2. Pathological causes of constipation

Disorders category	Specific disorders	
Endocrine/Metabolic	Panhypopituitarism Hypothyroidism Hypercalcemia Hypokalemia Pheochromocytoma	Acidosis Uremia Diabetes Porphyria
Peripheral neurologic	Hirschsprung's disease Ganglioneuromatosis Multiple sclerosis Paraneoplastic neuropathy	Chagas disease Paraplegia Scleroderma
Central nervous system	Depression Parkinson's disease Chronic psychosis Cerebrovascular accidents	Tumors Anorexia nervosa Meningocele Trauma to nervi erigentes or medulla
Extraluminal obstruction	Tumors Chronic volvulus	Hernias Proctoptosis
Luminal obstruction	Tumors Strictures Inflammatory stenosis	Ischemic stenosis Endometriosis
Muscular	Diverticular disease Systemic sclerosis Irritable colon syndrome	Myotonia dystrophia Chorionitis
Mucosal inflammatory	Proctosigmoiditis	
Rectal	Ulcerative proctitis Rectocele	
Anal	Arctation Anal fissure Abscesses	Hemorrhoids Mucosal prolapse Stenosis

Table 3. Classes and examples of drugs reported to cause constipation

---

Anesthetics (e.g. volatile anesthetics)
Antacids (e.g. calcium and aluminum compounds)
Antianorexia drugs (e.g. amphetamines)
Antianxiety drugs (e.g. benzodiazepines)
Antiarrhythmic drugs (e.g. verapamil)
Anticholinergics (e.g. atropine)
Anticonvulsants
Antidepressive agents (e.g. tricyclics, MAO inhibitors)
Antidiarrheal (e.g. loperamide)
Antihistamine drugs (e.g. anti-H_1)
Antihyperlipidemics (e.g. cholestyramine, colestipol)
Antihypertensive agents (e.g. clonidine, methyldopa, prazosin)
Antiinflammatory (e.g. indomethacin)
Antineoplastics (e.g. vinca derivatives, decarbazine)
Antipsychotic agents (e.g. phenothiazines)
Barium sulfate
Bismuth
Calcium channel blockers (e.g. verapamil)
Diuretics (e.g. benzothiadiazide, K-sparing diuretics)
Drugs for parkinsonism
Ganglionic blockers (e.g. guanethidine)
Hematinics (e.g. iron)
Laxatives, when chronically administered
Opiates

From Capasso and Di Carlo (1994).

constipation, but their mechanism is unknown. Other heavy metals such as barium and lead cause constipation (Brunton 1990; Racagni et al. 1986). Even laxatives, when used chronically, can lead to "rebound" constipation. This topic will be discussed further in the section on laxative abuse.

A rational treatment of functional constipation is that shown schematically in Table 4. The first objective is to reassure the patient, and explain the innocuity of the symptoms and the possibility of a successful return to normal bowel function by some training. The importance of following a regular pattern for bowel movements, for example after breakfast or dinner

Table 4. Treatment of functional constipation

- Educate and empathize with patients
- Increase consumption of a diet rich in fiber
- Increase water intake during the day
- Break the habit of taking laxatives

---

must be stressed. Finally, the advantage of appropriate exercises to strengthen the abdominal muscles should be pointed out. Another objective is to improve the diet by increasing the consumption of foods with a high fiber content. Table 5 lists some of the most common foods rich in fiber.

Table 5. Dietary fiber content of vegetables and breads

Food item	% Fiber
Apples	1.0
Artichokes	3.2
Asparagus	0.7
Bananas	0.6
Carrots	1.1
Dry figs	2.4
Dry plums	1.8
Fresh figs	1.7
Grapes	0.5
Green beans	1.4
Lettuce	0.6
Oranges	0.6
Peaches	0.6
Pears	1.4
Peas	2.2
Potatoes	0.4
Rye bread	1.2
Spinach	0.6
Tangerines	1.0
Tomatoes	0.6
White bread	0.5
Whole meal bread	1.2

From Capasso (1993).

Dietary fiber is one line of approach in an attempt to treat functional constipation. The laxative effects of bran have been known since antiquity, and today the benefits of fiber are still promoted. Shortly after the turn of this century, the physician-surgeon John Kellogg (Battle Creek, Michigan, of Kellogg cereal fame) promoted the benefits of a diet high in fiber, which will be dealt with in Chapter 5. However the value of some of these measures recommended for relief of constipation (increased fluid intake, physical activity, diet rich in fiber) is questionable (see Leng-Peschlow 1992). Thus serious cases of constipation require treatment with laxatives. Spastic constipation, as occurs in irritable bowel syndrome, is associated with slowed transit due to circular muscular contraction in the colon. Sometimes this condition is associated with pseudo-diarrhea. The most prominent symptom of spastic constipation is abdominal pain, which is alleviated by defecation. Anxiety and irritability also are usually present. In these cases supportive psychotherapy, anti-anxiety drugs, and a diet rich in fiber can be useful.

The use of laxatives is not restricted to the treatment of constipation. Laxatives are frequently used to ensure successful diagnostic studies of the gastrointestinal tract. Laxatives and large volumes of osmotic solutions are given to patients prior to sigmoidoscopy, barium enema examinations and colonoscopy (Binder 1988). Laxatives are also useful in some patients to decrease the effort required in defecation. As a result, patients recovering from recent myocardial infarction or during the postoperative period of abdominal or anorectal surgery are frequently given laxatives to prevent excess straining associated with defecation in order to prevent unnecessary cardiovascular stress in the former instance or perirectal discomfort in the latter. Laxatives are also employed to eliminate noxious material (food or drug) from the intestinal tract, or to remove parasites after administration of anthelmintic drugs. Laxatives are also used in the treatment of hepatic encephalopathy. Protein in the colon is often the source for increased ammonia production in patients with portal-systemic shunting. The laxative lactulose has been used to eliminate the excess ammonia in such patients.

The use of laxatives is unadvisable in patients undergoing oral therapy with some antibiotics, because these may cause sudden diarrhea (Capasso 1993), or in digitalized patients, because the effects of cardiac glucosides may be intensified and followed by signs of toxicity (Rondanelli et al. 1980; Newall et al. 1996). Finally, licorice, diuretics and corticosteroids may be synergistic with laxatives, increasing potassium loss (Refit 1996).

3. Role of Ion Transport in Laxative Action

3.1 Mucosal physiology relevant to laxatives

The principal function of the intestinal tract is to absorb water, electrolytes and nutrients from food. The quantity of water that reaches the colon in 24 h is about 9 L (Fig. 1). About 150 mL of this is found in the feces; 99% is absorbed, most by the jejunum, less by the ileum and about 15% by the colon (Binder 1989). Only a small volume (2 L) of this liquid is swallowed during the day, while most of it (7 L) is secreted throughout the digestive tract: saliva, 1.5 L; gastric juice, 2.5 L; bile, 0.5 L; pancreatic juice, 1.5 L; intestinal juice, 1.0 L). This liquid lubricates the stomach and intestine and eases the movement of the chyme through the gastrointestinal tract. The fluid also helps to remove residual food left in the intestinal passages (a washing function) and thus keeps bacteriological flora at physiological levels. Moreover, these secretions facilitate the movement of immunoglobulins from the crypts to sites more exposed to the lumen. When the absorption of fluid is excessive or when physiologic secretion is impaired, the feces become dehydrated and transit through the bowel may be slowed. On the other hand, when laxatives are given orally, fluid accumulates in the intestinal lumen, the rate of transit is increased and defecation is facilitated.

The mucosa of the small and large intestines is continually engaged in a process of moving ions and water from the lumen to the serosal interstitium and *vice versa*. It is really the difference between these concurrent fluxes of solutes and water that determines whether one is measuring absorption or secretion. The **accumulation of fluid in the intestinal lumen can occur from inhibition of absorption or stimulation of secretion.** Because what we measure experimentally is net absorption, comprised of the bidirectional movement of fluid, it is difficult to know which specific process has been affected. In 1960, Code et al. attempted to address this issue by characterizing the movement or transfer of water and other substances from the intestinal contents to the blood and *vice versa* as "insorption" and "exsorption", respectively. In conventional terms we would consider absorption to occur when the rate of insorption exceeds the rate of exsorption; when exsorption exceeds insorption, fluid accumulates in the lumen (Fig. 2). For convenience, and so not to confuse the reader, in this monograph we will use the terms "absorption" and "secretion", with the understanding that these processes merely describe the net result of simultaneous bidirectional ion fluxes (Nell and Rummel 1984).

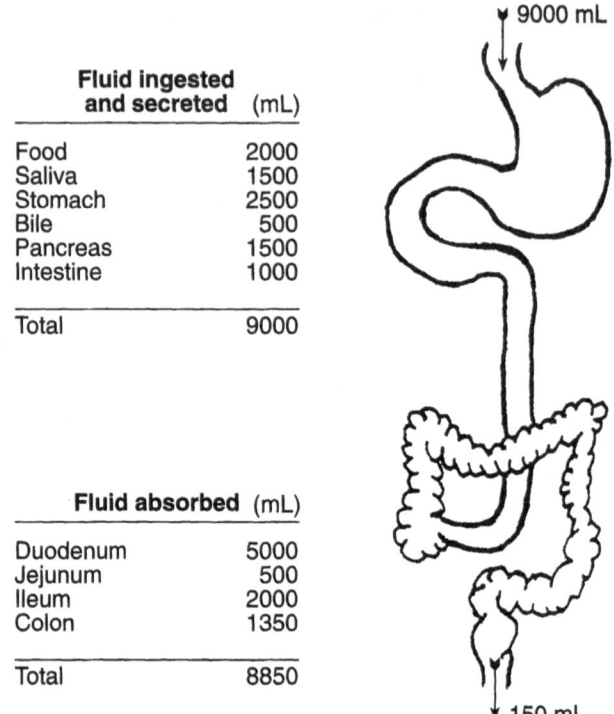

Fluid ingested and secreted	(mL)
Food	2000
Saliva	1500
Stomach	2500
Bile	500
Pancreas	1500
Intestine	1000
Total	9000

Fluid absorbed	(mL)
Duodenum	5000
Jejunum	500
Ileum	2000
Colon	1350
Total	8850

9000 mL

150 mL

Fig. 1. Fluid transport throughout the gastrointestinal tract. *Top*: fluid volumes entering the indicated segment. *Bottom*: fluid volumes absorbed in the segment

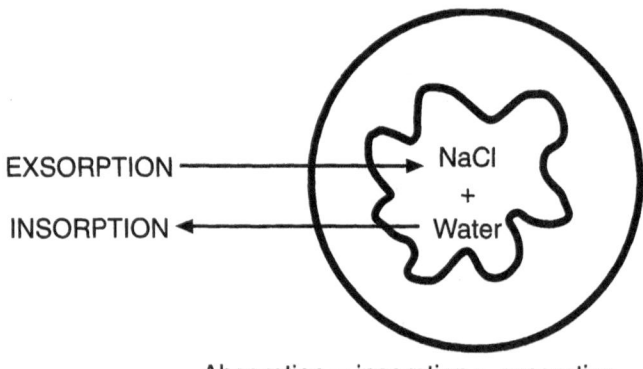

EXSORPTION

INSORPTION

NaCl + Water

Absorption = insorption > exsorption

Secretion = exsorption > insorption
(luminal accumulation)

Fig. 2. Functional definition of absorption and secretion (cross sectional view of intestine)

It should also be realized that secretion is a term usually reserved for a stimulated active process, such as occurs in response to cholera toxin (Binder 1977). The secretion and absorption of water and electrolytes take place in different types of epithelial cells: those which line the villi are believed to be primarily involved in absorption and those of the intestinal crypts are thought to be concerned with secretion. This separation between secretory and absorptive functions is largely a consequence of circumstantial evidence: disruption of villi does not decrease cholera toxin-induced fluid in the rabbit intestine (Roggin et al. 1972) and secretion induced by cholera toxin is evident only when crypt cell adenylyl cyclase is stimulated (De Jonge 1975). Cyclic adenosine monophosphate (cyclic AMP) inhibits absorption but does not cause secretion in the flounder gut, an epithelium devoid of crypt cells (Field et al. 1980).

The luminal (brush border) and basolateral (serosal) membranes of enterocytes represent two principal barriers to transepithelial electrolyte movement (Fig. 3). The intraluminal fluid is usually isotonic with plasma and contains Na^+ and Cl^- as the major cation and anion, respectively. Being more concentrated in the intestinal lumen than intracellularly, Na^+ enters the enterocyte passively. Once in the cell, Na^+ is actively transported across the basolateral (serosal or contraluminal) membrane through the action of Na^+, K^+-ATPase; water follows osmotically. In the ileum the absorption of Na^+ is coupled through an antiport

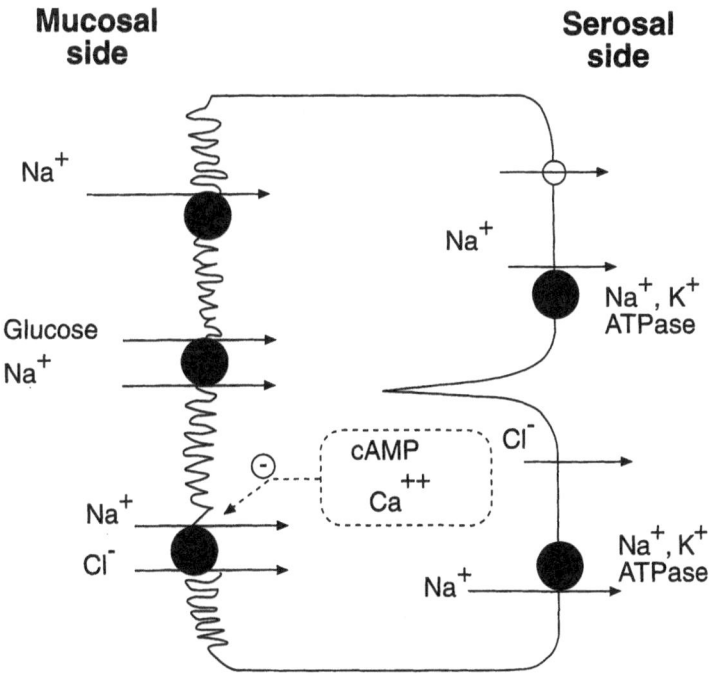

Fig. 3. Cellular mechanisms for transport of ions by intestinal epithelial cells

exchange mechanism to the secretion of H^+, and Cl^- is absorbed in exchange for HCO_3 (Turnberg et al. 1970). Secretion of water and electrolytes is a physiologic process that counterbalances absorption. The basal control of secretion may be regulated by neural and hormonal influences as well as by luminal factors such as bile salts. Water secreted in one part of the bowel may be absorbed subsequently in a more distal area. Thus, **a laxative effect can be produced by inhibition of absorption of fluid or stimulation of active secretion**. The result either way is the accumulation of fluid in the lumen. An increase in epithelial permeability (by creating a "leak") can also lead to luminal fluid accumulation. Some of the amphipathic (detergent) laxatives (e.g. long-chain fatty acids and bile acids) may act partly through such a mechanism. The substances that stimulate secretion act mainly through cyclic AMP, cyclic guanosine monophosphate (cyclic GMP), or calcium (Ca^{2+}) (Berridge 1983; Case et al. 1983; Powell 1983). Some of these substances (e.g. bile acids, fatty acids, enterotoxins) act luminally and others act through receptors (e.g. acetylcholine, prostaglandins, serotonin, vasoactive intestinal peptide) on the basolateral aspect of the enterocytes.

3.2 Second messengers

Until 1975, cyclic AMP was considered to be the major second messenger for stimulation of intestinal secretion. This was based largely on the fact that the secretagogues choleragen, theophylline, prostaglandins and vasoactive intestinal peptide (VIP) all increased tissue levels of cyclic AMP. Later it was demonstrated that serotonin, carbachol (a cholinergic agonist), and the calcium ionophore A 23187 induced intestinal secretion in a variety of experimental preparations (Donowitz and Welsh 1987). These agonists increased intracellular Ca^{2+} without affecting cyclic AMP levels, indicating that intracellular Ca^{2+} itself can mediate NaCl transport. The situation is complicated by the fact that cyclic AMP evokes Ca^{2+} release from mitochondria, and extracellular Ca^{2+} entry into the cytoplasm is accompanied by increased hydrolysis of membrane-associated phosphatidylinositol and polyphosphoinositides (Berridge 1983) which regulate Ca^{2+} homeostasis. Other experiments (Hardcastle and Wilkins 1970; Bolton and Field 1977;) have shown that intra- and extracellular Ca^{2+} are important in the effects of intestinal secretagogues and laxatives.

A variety of enzyme systems involved in metabolic functions and ion transport in epithelial and smooth muscle cells are Ca^{2+}-dependent (Table 6). Calcium exerts many of its actions through the calcium-dependent regulator protein calmodulin, present in epithelial cells. The involvement of calmodulin in the regulation of intestinal secretion is supported by the fact that inhibitors of calmodulin, such as trifluoperazine, prevent or inhibit secretion caused by secretagogues that raise intracellular Ca^{2+} (Donowitz and Welsh 1987).

Table 6. Enzyme systems sensitive to calcium

Adenylyl cyclase *	Myosin light chain kinase *
Ca^{2+}-ATPase	Na^+, K^+-ATPase
Cyclic nucleotide phosphodiesterases*	Nitric oxide synthase
Fructose 1,6 diphosphate	Phospholipases * (some)
Guanylyl cyclase *	Phosphofructokinase
Glycerol phosphate dehydrogenase	Phosphorylase b-kinase *
Glycogen synthase kinase	Pyruvate carboxylase
Isocitrate dehydrogenase	Pyruvate dehydrogenases
Lipases * (some)	Pyruvate kinase

* Through calmodulin

3.3 Autacoids and paracrine mediators

Several endogenous mediators that influence the regulation of fluid and secretion have been identified in the intestinal tract. Paracrine mediators are released by one cell and affect adjacent cells (e.g. histamine released by mucosal mast cells can stimulate secretion by the epithelial cells). Autacoids may be produced by the same cells that they act upon (e.g. prostaglandins), or they can act on cells other than those which produce them, by transport through the microcirculation (e.g. bradykinin).

Prostaglandins may be important in the physiological regulation of water and electrolyte transport in the gut. Their biosynthesis is initiated by non-specific stimulation such as membrane damage, or stimulation of cells by hormones, neurotransmitters or other autacoids (Rask-Madsen and Bukhave 1981). Prostaglandins are synthesized throughout the intestinal tract in the subepithelial layer subjacent to the secretory epithelial cells (Balaa and Powell 1986). Prostaglandins cause a greater elevation of cyclic AMP levels in crypt cells than in villus cells, suggesting that they produce active secretion secondary to cyclic AMP (Rask-Madsen and Bukhave 1983). However, *in vitro* studies have shown that prostaglandin concentrations 100-1000 times lower than those required to affect cyclic AMP activity evoke secretion. These findings, and the fact that serotonin and cholinergic agonists induce secretion by stimulating prostaglandin synthesis and increasing intracellular Ca^{2+} without affecting cyclic AMP, lead to the possibility that prostaglandins may also stimulate fluid secretion independently of cyclic AMP. Amphipathic laxatives, such as the long-chain fatty acid ricinoleic acid (from castor oil), may stimulate chloride secretion through prostaglandins (Fig. 4).

Another endogenous substance that can evoke electrolyte secretion in the intestine is platelet activating factor (PAF) (Benveniste et al. 1988; Mc

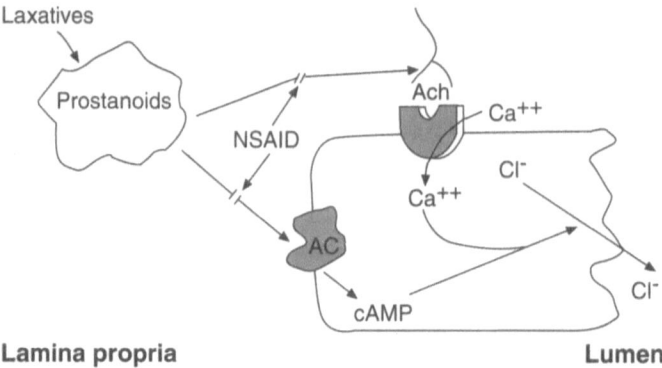

Fig. 4. Prostanoids as mediators of laxative-evoked intestinal secretion. *NSAID*, nonsteroid anti-inflammatory drugs; *Ach*, acetylcholine; *AC*, adenylyl cyclase. A potential mechanism only for certain laxatives; see text. (Modified from Gaginella 1990a)

Naughton and Gall 1991). It has been demostrated that administration of castor oil or diphenylmethane derivatives, but not senna, increases formation of PAF throughout the digestive tract (Pinto et al. 1989; Izzo et al. 1993) and causes diarrhea. However, at present no information exists about the effect of PAF on intestinal water accumulation and electrolyte secretion *in vivo* (Izzo 1996). It has been shown that PAF induces chloride secretion in the rat descending colon; this effect is independent of specific PAF receptors, probably because PAF is a small lipid molecule and may have direct effects on cell membranes independently of receptors (Buckley and Hoult 1989).

Recently it has also been shown that the L-arginine-NO pathway is involved in laxation induced by anthranoid and non anthranoid laxatives (Izzo et al. 1994, 1996b; Mascolo et al. 1994a, 1994b). However the precise involvement of PAF and NO in the mechanism of intestinal secretion and absorption is still unclear.

3.4 Neural control

The intestine contains an extensive network of intrinsic neurons and is richly innervated by extrinsic fibers of the sympathetic and parasympathetic branches of the autonomic nervous system. The majority of the nerves are confined to the large plexuses located in the submucosa and between the two muscle layers. The nervous control of gastrointestinal functions is thought to be mediated not only by adrenergic and cholinergic influences but also by peptidergic nerves and nerves that release nitric oxide (Brooks 1993).

Extrinsic adrenergic innervation projects abundant fibers to the crypt region. The effects of electrical stimulation of adrenergic nerves on electrolyte and intestinal fluid transport have been extensively studied both *in vitro* and *in vivo*. Some of these studies show that such stimulation increases the net uptake of Na$^+$ and Cl$^-$ and decreases anion secretion. Presumably such changes in electrolyte transport would lead to an increased fluid absorption or a decreased fluid secretion. These changes are a consequence of a direct alpha$_2$-adrenergic-receptor-mediated influence on the enterocyte, or an inhibition of a secretory influence. Cholinergic nerves also influence ion transport by the epithelium. Acetylcholine and synthetic muscarinic antagonists increase Cl$^-$ secretion (Gaginella 1990a). This can be considered a physiologic influence on intestinal ion transport, but excessive cholinergic activity may occur through vagal stimulation in irritable bowel syndrome and lead to nervous (i.e. neurogenic) diarrhea.

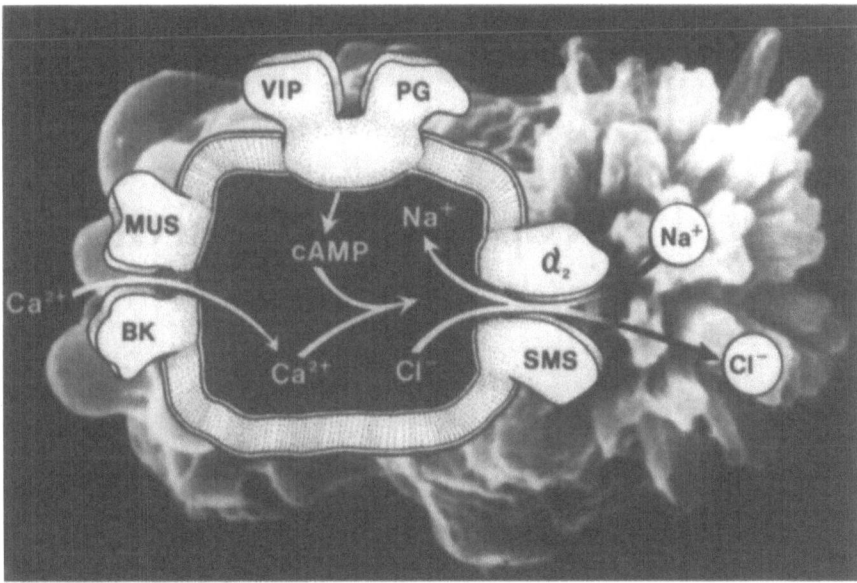

Fig. 5. Hypothetical involvement of neurohumoral receptors in epithelial cell transport of ions. The representation ignores origin (crypt, villus) of the cell. Muscarinic (*MUS*) and bradykinin (*BK*) receptors are present on the basolateral membranes of enterocytes and are linked to a calcium-mediated Cl$^-$ secretory response; although depicted as indicating Ca^{2+} influx, there may also be release of intracellular Ca^{2+}. Vasoactive intestinal polypeptide (*VIP*) and prostaglandin (*PG*) receptors in basolateral membranes evoke anion secretion through cyclic AMP (*cAMP*) as a second messenger. Alpha$_2$-adrenoceptors (α_2) and somatostatin (*SMS*) receptors promote cation movement from the luminal to the serosal aspects of the epithelium and/or inhibit cellular Cl$^-$ movement into the lumen. These two receptors effect similar changes in cellular function but are not identical. (With permission from Gaginella 1990b)

Immunohistochemistry has identified peptides that affect activity of the myenteric and submucosal nervous systems. These include substance P, VIP, enkephalins, somatostatin, and cholecystokinin. Of these, VIP best satisfies the conventional criteria for a neurotransmitter. It is located adjacent to the intestinal epithelium, in the crypts and villi, and it causes Cl^- secretion throughout the small intestine and colon (Gaginella et al. 1982). Figure 5 illustrates the hypothetical involvement of epithelial cell receptors for alpha-adrenoceptor agonists, muscarinic agonists, somatostatin and VIP. Receptors for autacoids, specifically prostaglandins and bradykinin, are shown. The figure also shows the relationship of these receptors to the second messengers calcium and cyclic AMP.

4. Intestinal Motility and Laxative Action

4.1 Synopsis of contractile physiology

The coordinated contractions of the smooth muscle of the intestine cause chyme to mix with intestinal fluids and to move aborally. Waves of contractions in the small intestine cause rhythmic segmentation, which rapidly mix the luminal contents. These nonpropulsive movements are accompanied by peristaltic movements, waves of contraction and relaxation that push the intestinal contents toward the colon (Weisbrodt 1987). Colonic motility also has segmenting-type movement; contraction and relaxation of the interhaustral rings, which churn the semi-liquid fecal material. By slowing down this process (colonic motility), absorption of water and electrolytes takes place until semi-solid feces (100-250 g per day) are formed in the most distal part of the colon. Retrograde contractions cause aberrant or slow transit, while the postprandial motor activity encourages movement of the intestinal contents towards the rectum.

Intestinal motility is controlled by myogenic, hormonal and nervous mechanisms (Christensen 1987). Cell membranes of the intestinal smooth muscle are polarized and depolarized with a regular rhythm. This basic electrical rhythm moves along the intestine with a frequency that varies from segment to segment. This myogenic activity is modulated by extrinsic autonomic neural input. There is also intrinsic neural control exerted by the activity of nerves in the myenteric and submucosal plexuses.

The motility of the small intestine is basically organized in two different patterns depending on the digestive state (Bueno et al. 1988; Sarna and Otterson 1988). The motility pattern, or the migrating motor complex (MMC), consists of contractions propagating in a coordinated fashion over longer distances, with the maximum frequency of contraction decreasing from duodenum to ileum. The MMC originates in the duodenum and migrates caudally to the ileocaecal junction; it has a duration of 6-8 min at any specific location and has a cyclic length of 120 min in man. In the MMC, three phases can be distinguished: phase 1 is a quiescent period; phase 2 is characterized by irregular motor activity which becomes more and more intense; phase 3 consists of bursts of rhythmic contractions migrating down the intestine (Bueno et al. 1988; Sarna and Otterson 1988). After feeding, the MMC is disrupted for 5-7 h and replaced by a continuous occurrence of irregular contractions; this period is characterized by a well-defined antroduodenal coordination (Bueno et al. 1988).

Autacoids and hormones can modify the contraction of the muscular wall of the intestine (Bardon and Deragnaucourt 1985; Bennett 1992). PAF, gastrin, motilin, and cholecystokinin stimulate intestinal contractions, whereas secretin, glucagon, VIP and nitric oxide inhibit them. The transit of the contents through the intestine may be delayed, not only by neural disturbances but also by pathophysiology. A delay in transit may be aggravated by the dehydration of the feces, leading to constipation. Also, an increase in tone of intestinal smooth muscle (as produced by opiates) could reduce transit time and reduce fluid volume of the luminal contents. Distension of the gut can evoke secretion through a reflex mechanism (Caren et al. 1974; Itasaka et al. 1992). Reflex secretion also helps to remove residual debris from the intestinal lumen and thus helps to keep bacteria to a low level.

Contrary to common belief, transit through the intestine is decreased when circular muscle motility is increased because flow through the lumen is restricted. This can be the case in constipated patients and is the major pharmacologic effect of morphine and other opiates on the bowel. Alternatively, when measurements indicate that the circular muscle is contracting less frequently or less forcefully, the flow (transit) increases and laxation can result (Gullikson and Bass 1984). Figure 6 illustrates this concept.

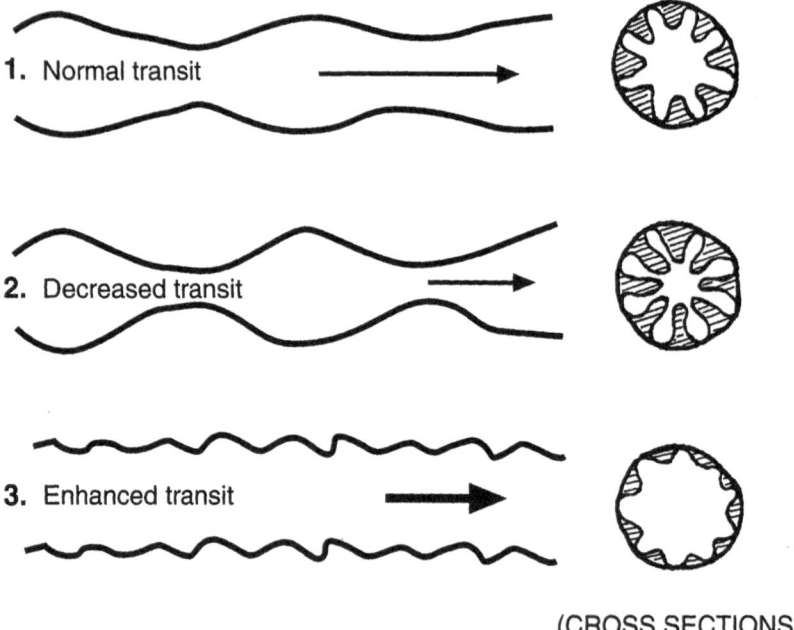

(CROSS SECTIONS)

Fig. 6. Motility (circular muscle activity) as related to reduced and enhanced transit. 1. normal; 2. increased activity as with morphine (constipation); 3. decreased activity as may occur with castor oil. (From Gaginella 1977)

4.2 Defecation

The feces reach the rectum only when defecation is about to begin. The filling of the rectum and its distension, which results from the pressure, bring about a series of reflexes. In succession these are relaxation of the anal sphincters, contact of the feces with the anal canal, contraction of the external and internal sphincters, and defecation. The expulsion of the feces is promoted by an increase in intra-abdominal pressure, brought about voluntarily by the contractions of the muscles of the abdominal wall and of the diaphragm.

Defecation is controlled by the central nervous system through the lumbar and sacral zones of the spinal cord. The lumbar tract innervates the muscular wall of the rectum (inhibitory effect) and the intestinal smooth muscle sphincters (stimulatory effect). The sacral fibers innervate the muscular wall of the rectum (stimulatory effect) as well as internal sphincters (inhibitory effect) and the externally striated muscle sphincters. The former sphincter controls the containment of the feces; the latter controls their expulsion.

5. Laxatives of Botanical Origin

5.1 Anthraquinones

The principal *anthraquinones* are found in *Rhamnus frangula* and *R. purshiana, Aloe ferox, A. barbadensis, A. succotrina, A. vera* and *A. africana, Rheum palmatum* and *R. officinale, Cassia acutifolia* and *C. angustifolia*. The common name for the last group is Indian or African senna; these plants contain sennosides with anthranoid structures like those found in the *Rhamnus* and *Aloe* plants. The anthraquinones usually occur in nature as glycoside derivatives of anthracene. The glycosides behave like pro-drugs, liberating the aglycone that acts as the laxative. Figures 7 and 8 show the principal glycoside forms of natural anthraquinones and their metabolism to the active aglycones. The metabolism takes place in the colon (Fig. 9), where bacterial glycosidases remove D-glucose or L-rhamnose (Longo 1980; Hattori et al. 1982; Dreessen and Lemli 1988). Germ-free animals do not have a laxative response to orally administered anthraquinones. The products obtained are poorly absorbed and act by evoking secretory and motility changes in the colon (Hardcastle and Wilkins 1970; Garcia-Villar et al. 1980; Leng-Peschlow 1980; Beubler and Kollar 1985; Leng-Peschlow 1986; Frexinos et al. 1989; de Witte et al. 1991). The effect on secretion is probably the consequence of exaggerated intestinal production of prostaglandins and of other autacoids (Beubler and Juan 1979; Capasso et al. 1986; Autore et al. 1990a, 1990b; Nijs et al. 1991). Likewise the effect on motility is at least in part due to a release of prostaglandins and other autacoids (Autore et al. 1984; Capasso et al. 1986; Staumont et al. 1988; Yagi et al. 1988). However, it is not proven that prostaglandins have a role in the laxative action of senna (Mascolo et al. 1988a, 1988b). The stimulatory motility effects *in vivo* can be blocked by local anesthetics, suggesting that the submucosal nerves are activated by mucosal contact with anthraquinones (Hardcastle and Wilkins 1970). However, several *in vitro* studies show inhibition of contractility (motility) of the intestinal muscle upon contact with these drugs (Latven et al. 1952; Gullikson and Bass 1984; Odenthal and Ziegler 1988).

The mechanism of action of anthraquinone aglycones includes inhibition of small intestinal and colonic NaCl absorption and stimulation of Cl⁻ secretion. A common aglycone anthraquinone is 1,8-dihydroxyquinone, also known as danthron. The inhibitory effect that the aglycones have on absorption can be explained by inhibition of Na^+, K^+-ATPase (Wanitschke

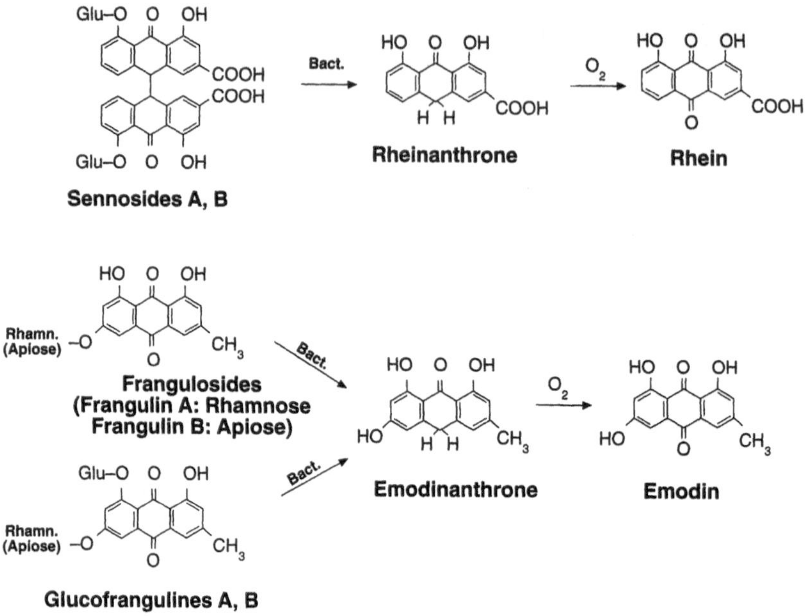

Fig. 7. Metabolism of sennosides, frangulosides and glucofrangulines to the aglycones rhein and emodin

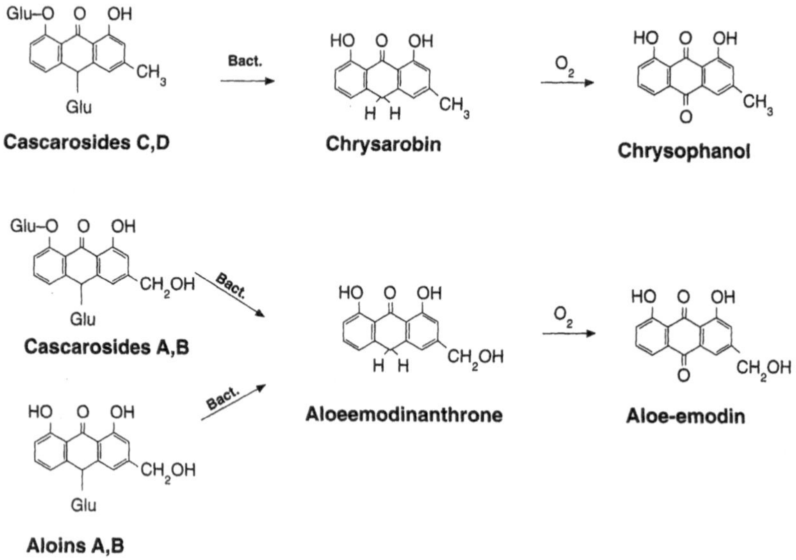

Fig. 8. Metabolism of cascara glycosides and aloins to the aglycones chrysophanol and aloe-emodin

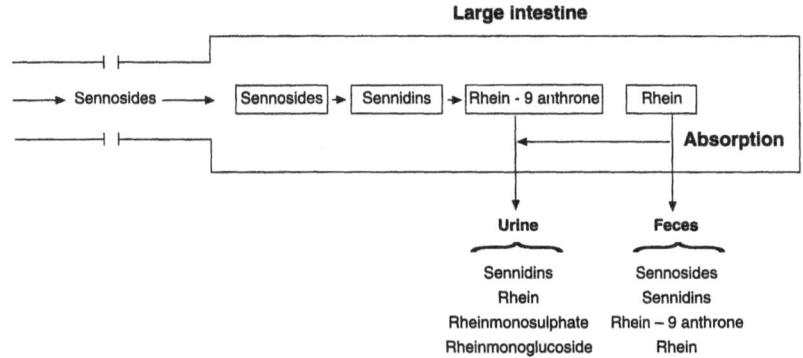

Fig. 9. Metabolism, distribution and excretion of sennosides

1980; Ishii et al. 1990) but the secretion is apparently not due to cyclic AMP or calcium (Donowitz and Welsh 1987). Mucosal permeability changes are probably not involved (Leng-Peschlow 1992; Mascolo et al. 1992; Milner et al. 1992). Chronic treatment with anthranoids in high doses reduces VIP and somatostatin levels in the rat colon (Tzavella et al. 1995). This may represent a pharmacological effect of the anthranoids or cell injury through a decreased synthesis or increased breakdown of these peptides. Anthranoid laxatives induce subepithelial congestion of capillaries and epithelial alterations (Spiessens et al. 1991). These findings are in disagreement with those of other authors who found no mucosal abnormalities (Douthwaith and Goulding 1957; Dufour and Gendre 1988; Rudolph and Mengs 1988) and no alterations in parameters of intestinal physiology after short- or long-term treatment with senna preparation (Dubecq and Palmade 1974; Mahon and Palmade 1974).

Recently it has been shown that senna increases constitutive calcium-dependent nitric oxide (NO) synthase while cascara also induces calcium-independent NO synthase (Izzo et al. 1997). These results, and the fact that senna does not increase PAF formation (Fig. 10) throughout the digestive tract (Pinto et al. 1989; Capasso et al. 1993; Izzo et al. 1993), nor the intraluminal release of acid phosphatase, a marker of cellular injury (Capasso et al. 1993), indicates that some anthraquinones are well tolerated. The effect on nitric oxide could influence intramural neural and smooth muscle activity in such a way as to cause laxation.

Nausea and colic pain associated with the use of large doses of crude anthraquinone drugs are prevented by the use of lower doses or purified glycosides. The laxative action of the anthraquinones occurs 6-12 h after oral ingestion. The side effects include discoloration of the urine, reversible melanosis of the colon (Wittoesch et al. 1958) and hemorrhoid congestion. No changes in serum electrolyte levels were found with recommended doses of anthranoids, in particular sennosides (Heiny 1976; Rosprich 1980). A review article by Illingworth (1953) let us believe for years that active anth-

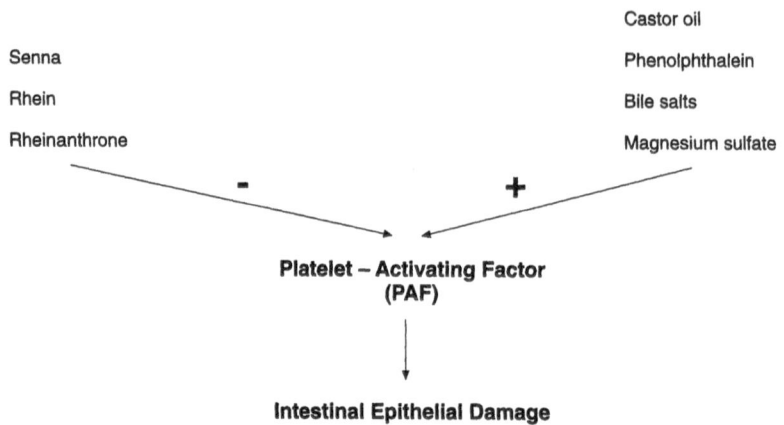

Senna   Castor oil

Rhein   Phenolphthalein

Rheinanthrone   Bile salts

                                         Magnesium sulfate

−   +

Platelet – Activating Factor
(PAF)

Intestinal Epithelial Damage

Fig. 10. Activation of PAF biosynthesis by laxatives; + activation; – no activation

ranoid could appear in the milk during lactation in amounts sufficient to affect the nursing infant. Instead, several clinical studies have shown that the treatment of lactating mothers with anthranoids like senna does not carry a risk of producing a laxative effect in the infant (Duncan 1957; Baldwin 1963; Werthmann and Krees 1973; Faber and Strenge-Hesse 1988; Cameron et al. 1988). Clinical studies also indicate that treatment with senna does not involve any increased risk during pregnancy or for the fetus (Wager and Melosh 1958; Scott 1965; Mahon and Palmade 1974; Bauer 1977). On the contrary, senna seems the laxative of choice in pregnancy and during feeding (Gattuso and Kamm 1994). In addition, no experimental or clinical evidence for an abortifacient action is found in the literature on aloe (Vago 1969; Fingl 1975), although it had been considered abortifacient in folk medicine (Prochnow 1911).

Anthraquinone - containing herbal drugs are currently recommended for short-term treatment (1-2 weeks) of atonic constipation, some cases of acute constipation and before endoscopy of the gastrointestinal tract; they are not advisable for spastic constipation. Anthranoids combined with fiber (senna-fiber combination) are also effective and well tolerated for chronic constipation in elderly patients (Passmore et al. 1993). It is enough to give elderly patients a senna-fiber combination once or twice a week to restore normal motility in the large intestine and to normalize stool consistency (the production of soft or liquid stools should be avoided). The senna-fiber combination has been found more effective than lactulose and less costly (Passmore et al. 1993). Also a combination senna-psyllium (Agiolax®) is more efficient than lactulose in treating constipation in geriatric long-stay patients (Kinnunen et al. 1993). These drugs should not be used for treating constipation associated with proctitis or hemorrhoids, or by women during menstruation.

Free anthraquinones are known to have also such diverse effects as anti-tumour properties (emodin), antibacterial and antifungal activities (aloe-emodin) and bactericidal action against *Bacteroides fragilis*, a bacterium responsable of hepatic and gallbladder diseases (Nishioka 1985).

5.1.1 Cascara

Cascara consists of the bark (Fig. 11) of the trunk or branches of the *Rhamnus purshiana De Candolle* (family Rhamnaceae), a shrub that grows along the Pacific coast of North America (Fig. 11). The shrub is 4-10 m high, with eliptical leaves dented on the edges, and flowers gathered in corymbs at the axil. The bark should be collected at least one year prior to use (to allow the reduced emodin - type glycosides to be oxidized to monomeric forms which exhibit a milder cathartic activity) at the beginning of the spring and continuing until the rainy season starts. Once dried, the bark becomes rounded in a pipe-form which is curved or almost flat, with a thickness of 1-4 mm and a variable length and width. At times it splits into little fragments almost uniformly flat.

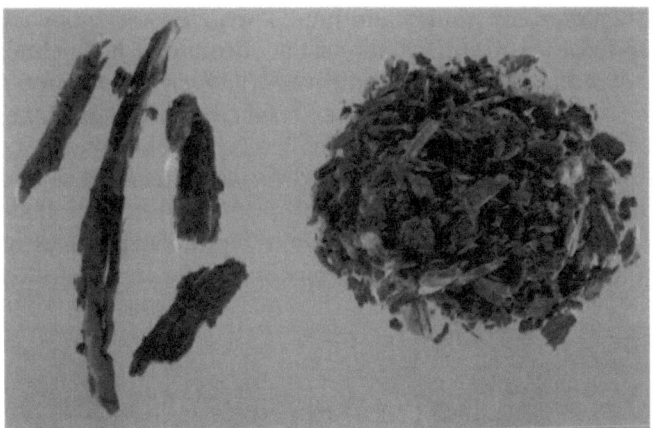

Fig. 11. Cascara

Cascara owes its action to a mixture of active compounds consisting largely of cascarosides A, B, C and D, with other anthraquinone glycosides in minor amounts. Cascara must contain not less than 7% total hydroxyanthracene derivatives calculated as cascaroside A on a dried basis. Because of its mild action, cascara produces weak side effects (griping). Only very small amounts of the active ingredients are secreted in breast milk, so this drug can be used by nursing mothers without adverse effects on the infant (Bennett 1988). Cascara is used in the form of extract, fluid extract, aromatic fluid extract (a 5 ml dose usually causes laxation) and powder (1 g in capsule form). However, the bitter taste is reduced by treating cascara extracts with magnesium oxide or alkaline earths; this treatment also reduces the activity of the extracts. Cascara tea is not popular because of its extremely bitter taste (Tyler 1994). Preparations containing purified anthranol glycosides (casanthranol) from cascara are also available (the adult dose is 30 mg). The laxative action occurs after about 8-12 h, and so it generally is taken before retiring. The drug is an ingredient of several over-the-counter (OTC) laxatives (Tyler et al. 1988).

A preparation containing cascara, boldo, inositol and cyanocobalamin has been used in the treatment of constipation in geriatric patients (Colombo 1994). Such a preparation increases significantly evacuations, improves asthenia and anorexia and reduces transaminase.

5.1.2 Frangula

This drug is derived from the bark of *Rhamnus frangula* Linne (family Rhamnaceae) (Fig. 12), a shrub 3-5 m high that grows in southern Central Europe and western Asia. Like cascara, frangula should be collected one year prior to use, preferably in May and June. The dried bark appears as a single or double pipe form which is almost flat or rounded. Its thickness is from 0.5 to 2 mm and its length and width vary. The bark has a brown-greyish surface. Its laxative effect is due to the presence of anthraquinone derivatives, particularly glucofrangulins A and B and frangulins A and B. Frangula must contain not less than 6% total hydroxyanthracene derivatives calculated as glucofrangulin A on a dried basis. Frangula is comparable to cascara in its relatively gentle laxative action; it is popular in its native Europe but less so in the United States. It is used in the form of fluid extract (see

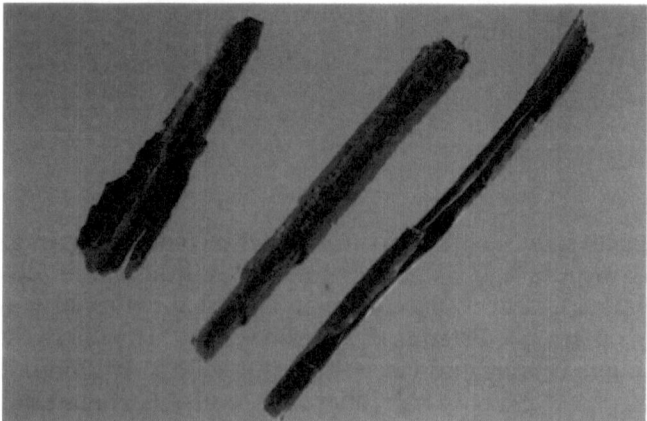

Fig. 12. Frangula

cascara) but it is also possible to consume the powdered bark (1 g) in capsule form. The laxative action occurs after about 10-12 h.

Preparations from the ripe fruits (dried) of *R. catharticus* Linne are also used for their cathartic action.

5.1.3 Aloe

The drug consists of the solid residue obtained by evaporating the latex (juice) which drains from the transversally cut leaves of several species of aloe (family Liliaceae), especially *Aloe barbadensis* Miller (*A. vera* Linne), known in commerce as Curaçao aloe, or *A. ferox* Miller, and hybrids of these species with *A. africana* Miller and *A. spicata* Burm, known in commerce as Cape aloe (Fig. 13). Curaçao aloe grows in the West Indian islands of Curaçao while Cape aloe grows in South Africa and Kenya. These plants have woody stems which have a height of a few decimeters. At the end of these grow a rosette of fleshy pointed leaves, from which rise a crown with flowers. Aloe is obtained from specialized cells (pericycle tubules) that occur at the border of the outer and inner cortical layers of the mesophyll located just beneath the epidermis of the leaves of the aloe plant. The yellow latex found there, when condensed to dryness, becomes a shiny mass, like broken glass of a yellow-greenish to red-black color. This drug is different from the colorless muci-laginous mass (*aloe gel*) obtained from the parenchyma tissue making up the central portion of the aloe leaf. Aloe gel contains mucilage, polysaccharides (acemannan, betamannan), crude aloin oil and resin as well as fat, protein and fiber (Hormann and Korting, 1994); it is an antiinflammatory and a wound-healing agent and never must be confused with aloe latex, the laxative drug.

The anthraquinone glycosides aloins A and B (barbaloin and iso-barba-

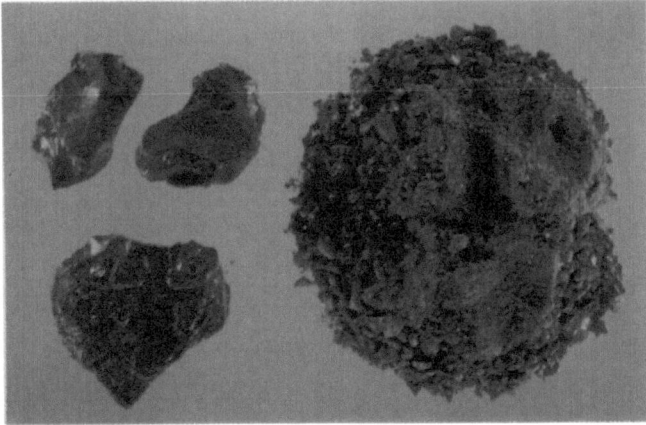

Fig. 13. Aloe

loin respectively) account for the laxative action of aloe. In addition to aloins (10-30%), aloe contains a volatile oil and large amounts of a resinous material (16-63%). Taken in doses of 0.25 g, aloe causes laxative action after 6-12 h with loose bowel movements accompanied by abdominal pain. Among the anthraquinones, aloe possesses the most potent action: it is less employed now because it tends to cause griping and has an effect persisting over several days (Grindlay and Reynolds 1986). Excessive doses or a prolonged use may cause nephrytis, gastritis, vomiting and diarrhea with elimination of mucus and blood. It should be used with caution in patients with nephropathy. It is seldomly prescribed alone and its activity is increased when administered with small quantities of soap or alkaline salts.

The aloe plant also produces antiseptic agents (lupeol, salicylic acid, urea nitrogen, cinnamic acid, phenol, sulfur), antiinflammatory fatty acids (cholesterol, campesterol, ß-sitosterol), glycoproteins (aloctin A and B) and some prostanoids. A whole leaf aloe extract, deprived of aloin (a cathartic), taken internally and externally is a therapeutically effective product, particularly in the areas of inflammation, wound healing and cancer (Capasso, personal communication).

5.1.4 Rhubarb

Rhubarb laxative consists of the dried rhizome and root of *Rheum palmatum* Linne, *R. officinale* Baillon (Polygonaceae) or of related species (*R. emodi* Wallich, *R. webbianum* Royl) or hybrids grown in China (Chinese rhubarb) or in India, Pakistan or Nepal (Indian or Himalayan rhubarb). *R. palmatum* and *R. officinale* are perennial herbaceous plants, 1-3 m tall with large heart-shaped or rounded leaves. The anthraquinones are especially concentrated in the rhizome which is collected in autumn or spring. The pie-

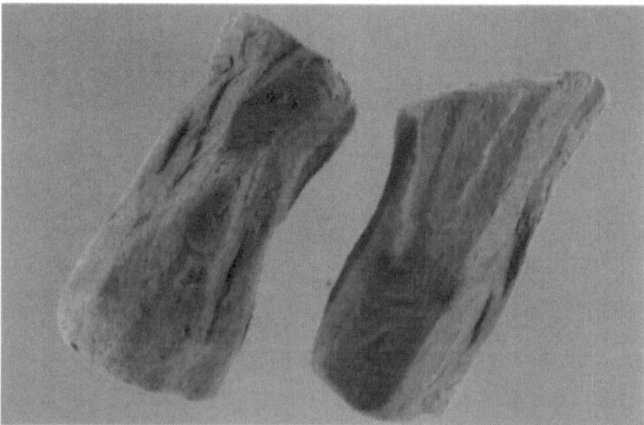

Fig. 14. Rhubarb

ces are of various forms (cylindrical, oval, rounded or with a convex surface) and sizes (5-15 mm in length and 4-10 mm in diameter) (Fig. 14).

Rhubarb contains sennosides A-F with purgative properties [the laxative action is drastic (Robbers et al. 1996)], a considerable quantity of tannin (rhatannin), lindleyin, isolindleyin and the same stilbenes as found in the root of *Polygonum multiflora*. This drug, like aloe, is much more potent than cascara or senna (Tyler 1994). Its use almost always causes intestinal griping or colic. However, a laxative action without abdominal pain is caused by a dose of 0.5-2 g. The preparations most used are tinctures, infusions and fluid extracts. Frequent use is not recommended (Beck and Beck, 1982).

Rhubarb is also effective in decreasing blood urea nitrogen and has anti-inflammatory and analgesic properties (Nishioka 1985).

5.1.5 Senna

Of all the anthranoid laxatives, the most used is certainly senna. Senna consists of the leaves and pods of *Cassia acutifolia* Delile, known in commerce as Alexandria senna, or of *Cassia angustifolia* Vahl, known as Tinnevelly senna (Fig. 15). These bushes (shrubs) of the family of Leguminosae (family Fabaceae according to others) are native to Egypt (*C. acutifolia* grows wild near the Nile River), the Middle East (Somalia and Arabian peninsula), and India. They grow to 20-60 cm high and are characterised by paripinnate compound leaves, arranged in clusters of 4-7 small leaves opposite each other, and pod-like fruits. Taxonomists now group both of these species together under the scientific name *Senna alexandrina* Miller. The leaves are green-greyish in color with an elongated and pointed form. The fruit is blackish, elongated, flat and kidney-shaped. Senna is harvested in April and in September.

Dianthrone glycosides, particularly sennosides A, A_1, B, C, D, and G, together with other anthraquinone derivatives, account for the laxative action of senna. Although senna is not as mild in its actions as cascara or fran-

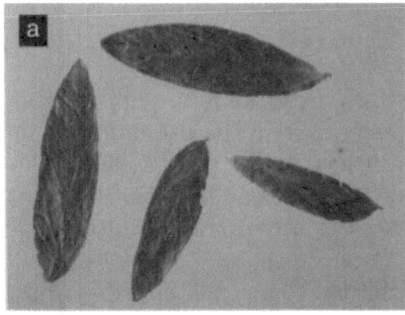
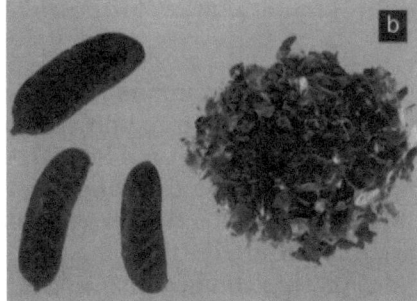

Fig. 15 a, b. Senna: leaves (a) and pods (b)

gula, it is more widely used because it is considerably cheaper. Syrup and fluid extracts made from the leaves or pods are available. These preparations (8 mL syrup, 2 mL fluid extract, or 2 g senna) usually produce a single bowel evacuation within 6 h. A bitter-tasting tea can be prepared from 0.5-2 g of senna; however some prefer a beverage prepared by soaking senna in cold water for 10-12 h and then straining. Such a preparation is more active than the hot tea as it contains more sennosides and will contain less resinous material (Wichtl 1984). Crystalline senna glycosides (sennosides) are also available; they are more stable, more reliable and safer than the preparations of crude senna (Mc Clure Browne et al. 1957; Hietala et al. 1987). The usual dose of sennosides is 12-36 mg. In drug preparations senna is combined with various substances.

5.2 Castor oil

Castor oil, from the seeds of *Ricinus communis* Linne (family Euphorbieceae), has been used as a laxative for centuries (Gaginella and Phillips 1975). Use of the *Ricinus* plant by Egyptians is recorded in the Ebers Papyrus. The Aztecs also utilized a variety of the plant for medicinal purposes. The 1788 edition of the London Pharmacopeia and the Edinburgh New Dispensatory of 1797 make reference to castor oil. In the 19th Century it was ironically used in dysentery because it was thought to act by providing an oily coating over the mucosa. The active component of castor oil was identified in 1890 as ricinoleic acid, an 18-carbon Δ 9-10 mono-unsaturated fatty acid, hydroxylated at the C-12 position (Fig. 16). Ricinoleic acid is present in castor oil as the triglyceride.

$$\underset{|}{\text{OH}}$$
$$CH_3(CH_2)_5CHCH_2CH=CH(CH_2)_7COOH$$

Fig. 16. Chemical formula of ricinoleic acid

Castor oil is used commonly to evacuate the bowel prior to surgery or radiologic, sigmoidoscopic and proctoscopic procedures. The usual dose is 15-60 mL. The oil is also used for total colonic evacuation prior to labor. The unpleasant odor and taste of castor oil can be hidden a bit by emulsifying it with peppermint into a creamy mixture or simply stirring it into orange juice prior to administration.

After oral ingestion, castor oil mixes with bile and pancreatic enzymes which liberate ricinoleic acid. Some ricinoleic acid is absorbed from the gastrointestinal tract but most remains in the intestine, where it forms ricinoleate salts with sodium and potassium. These amphipathic molecules act as soaps (surfactants) at the mucosal surface. Contrary to popular belief, castor oil is not an irritant to the intestinal lining and it does not stimulate the coordinated movement of gastrointestinal propulsion. Contractility *in vitro* of longitudinal muscle from the small intestine of rodents is not stimulated but is depressed by ricinoleate (Stewart et al. 1975a,b). Therefore, it is not appropriate to classify castor oil as a stimulant laxative.

Modern experimental techniques have made it possible to investigate in considerable detail the mechanism of action of ricinoleate on the mucosa and smooth muscle of the gut. The rhythmic pattern of electrical activity which drives the coordinated movement of intraluminal contents through the bowel is disrupted by castor oil (Gullikson and Bass 1984). Exposure of the intestinal mucosa to ricinoleic acid (5 mM or greater) causes inhibition of water and electrolyte absorption from the jejunal and ileal lumen, increasing the fluidity of the contents. This concentration can be achieved in the lower bowel after a normal therapeutic dose of castor oil (30 mL). Coupled with the effects of ricinoleate on intestinal smooth muscle, this causes an increase in transit through the small intestine, further reducing the time for absorption to take place. Ricinoleate also inhibits absorption and stimulates secretion by the colonic mucosa (Phillips and Gaginella 1977).

At concentrations from 2 to 10 mM, ricinoleate has several actions that may account for its anti-absorptive/pro-secretory effect. It inhibits the sodium-potassium ATPase, increases permeability of the intestinal epithelium, produces a cytotoxic effect on isolated enterocytes and inhibits epithelial cell mitochondrial metabolism (see Gaginella 1990a). It also may stimulate (or inhibit) epithelial cell adenylyl cyclase, and release prostaglandins, kinins and platelet activating factor (Autore et al. 1990b; Capasso et al. 1985a; Capasso et al. 1992; Gaginella 1990a). Most recently, nitric oxide has been claimed to contribute to the laxative action of castor oil (Mascolo et al. 1993). Ricinoleic acid may act as a calcium ionophore (Maenz and Forsyth 1982), increasing the influx of extracellular calcium, thus activating calmodulin-dependent secretory mechanisms.

All of these effects might be due to the mucosal injury and enhanced cell membrane permeability produced by ricinoleate (Bretagne et al. 1981; Beubler and Juan 1979; Cline et al. 1979). In the colon ricinoleate causes loss of surface epithelial cells when perfused at 10 mM (Fig. 17). However, it recently has been demonstrated to be possible to dissociate the laxative effect of castor oil from intestinal mucosal damage (Capasso et al. 1994). These findings suggest that laxation and mucosal damage are independent. The relationship between nitric oxide and PAF in castor oil-induced mucosal injury has also been studied (Mascolo et al. 1996). The results lead to speculation that the endogenous production of PAF and NO are in a fine balance, and a suppression in NO production could result in an increase in PAF biosynthesis which could lead to mucosal injury. A summary of the multiple effects of

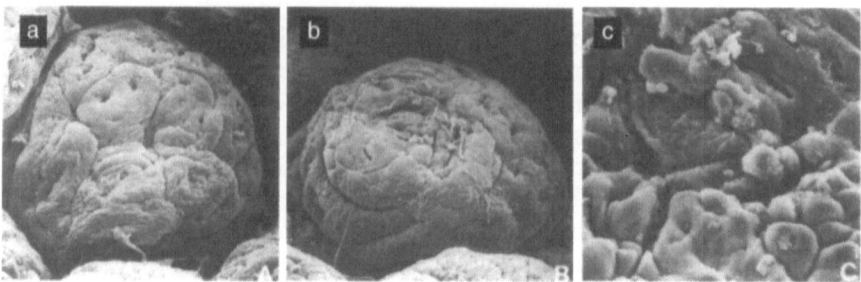

Fig. 17 a-c. Effect of perfusion of 10 mM ricinoleate through rabbit colon. Scanning electron micrograph of rabbit colon perfused with 5 mM sodium ricinoleate. **a** a control tissue (x 300); **b** a low power (x 400) view of the mucosal surface; **c** an enlarged view (x 1.900) of the damaged area on the surface. Note in **b** the loss of ephitelial cells and the presence of debris in the central portion of the view; this is more clearly seen in **c**. The mucosal injury is probably responsible for the release of prostanoids and the subsequent enhancement of cyclic adenosine monophosphate levels observed in some instances after exposure of the mucosa to ricinoleate or other surfactant laxatives. (From Gaginella 1990a)

castor oil (ricinoleate) on fluid accumulation in the intestinal lumen is given in Table 7.

The effects are compared with those produced by other laxatives to be discussed in subsequent sections of this monograph.

Castor oil is usually administered on an empty stomach and acts within

Table 7. Intraluminal water and electrolyte accumulation as related to the mechanism of action of common laxatives[a]

	Na^+, K^+, ATPase inhibition	Cyclic AMP stimulation	Ca^{+2} involved	Increased permeability or mucosal injury	Autacoid release	PAF release	NO release
Castor oil	yes	yes	yes	yes	yes	yes	yes
Phenolphthalein	yes	yes	not tested	yes	yes	yes	yes
Bisacodyl	yes	yes	not tested	yes	yes	yes	yes
Oxyphenisatin	yes	no	not tested	yes	yes/no	not tested	not tested
Anthraquinones	yes	no	yes/no	no	yes	no	yes
DSS	yes	yes	not tested	yes	yes	yes	not tested
Picosulfate	yes	yes	not tested	yes/no	yes	yes	not tested

[a] The data are derived mostly from animal experiments; these effects are not proven to occur in human subjects.

PAF, platelet activating factor; NO, nitric oxide; DSS, dioctyl sulfosuccinate.

2-6 h. The common side effect from castor oil is intestinal discomfort. Long-term use (abuse) can adversely change normal motility of the bowel and may result in electrolyte imbalance.

5.3 Olive and other vegetable oils

The fixed oil expressed from olives has been used as a laxative. Olive oil is comprised mostly of oleic acid, a 18-carbon mono-unsaturated aliphatic fatty acid. Part of the mechanism by which olive oil produces a laxative effect probably involves oleic acid acting upon the mucosa in a manner similar to ricinoleic acid, which comes from castor oil (all above). The use of olive oil as a laxative is quite uncommon but, nevertheless, when taken in an oral dose of 30 mL it is capable of acting as such. Olive oil has the disadvantage of being absorbed and therefore contributes to a calorie intake which may not be advisable for obese patients. Olive oil is obtained from the ripe drupe of *Olea europaea* (family Oleaceae) by pressure extraction at a cold temperature. It is a clear liquid, pale yellow or greenish-yellow, with the characteristic smell and taste of the olive. It begins to thicken when cooled to 10°C, and at about 0°C it forms a buttery mass.

Other vegetable oils with laxative effects are almond oil and peanut oil. The former is a fatty oil obtained under cold pressure of the ripe seed of *Prunus amigdalus*, of the dulcis variety (family Rosaceae). It is a pale yellow liquid, very fluid almost without smell and with a sweetish taste. Peanut oil is a fatty, refined oil, obtained from the seeds of one or more cultivated varities of *Arachis hypogaea* (family Leguminosae). It is a colorless or pale yellow liquid with a pleasant and characteristic smell and taste.

5.4 Dietary fiber - Bulk-forming laxatives

The benefits of dietary fiber in maintaining a healthy colon and normal bowel movements have been promulgated in Western society since the 1920s (Kellogg 1921; Schmidt and Von Noorden 1936). Additional health benefits have been ascribed to dietary fiber, as referenced by Bennett and Cerda (1996). Nevertheless, others during this same time period suggested that a low residue diet was best in order to rest an unstable colon (Tidmarsh 1936). It became clear by the late 1930s that constipation could be treated by taking advantage of the gentle laxative effects of dietary fiber (Kantor and Cooper 1937). The amount of fiber normally consumed in the diet varies greatly throughout the world, with Americans, British and Europeans generally having a low amount of indigestible residue as a part of their diet. The average British diet contains about 12 g dietary fiber compared to 60 g in the average African diet. As Thompson (1980) so cleverly put it, "English researchers, in the best tradition of Doctor Livingstone and Mungo Park, have documented stool weight and transit time in western and developing societies. Ugandan villagers, ingesting wholly unrefined food, produce an average of 470 grams of stools per day. On the other hand, British naval personnel, consuming a diet representative of British cuisine, produce an average of 104 grams daily. Even African children produce stools three times as large as those of sailors in the Royal Navy. The Ugandans have a gastrointestinal transit time of 36 hours as opposed to 83 hours for the fiber-deficient British tars. Canadians and Americans did not participate in these gastrointestinal olympics, but data from our unit suggests that the average Ottawa stool weight is 130 grams per day".

Fiber is defined as undigested soluble and insoluble residue remaining after a meal, consisting of pectin, gums and mucilages, cellulose, hemicellulose, polysaccharides and lignin (Table 8). Many of these insoluble polymers are hydrophilic and increase the bulk of the stool by attracting and retaining water. However, the capacity of fiber to retain water is not directly correlated with its effectiveness as a laxative (Gullikson and Bass 1984). Cellulose is a long unbranched molecule containing 1,4-β-D-glucose, which the enzymes of the human intestine cannot digest. Hemicellulose is similar to cellulose except that it contains a variety of hexose and pentose sugars in addition to glucose. It is believed to have the greatest water retaining capacity of the indigestible fibers. Lignin is present in plants, particularly the stems and leaves. Pectins are also derived from plants but are present in the skins and pulp of citrus fruits and apples. They form a gel-like material in the presence of water. Similarly, various plant gums and mucilages retain water but tend to become slippery and less thick than the cellulose-type residues.

Table 8. Dietary vegetable fibers

Substance	Characteristics
Cellulose	Straight chain, 1,4-β-D-glucose, mol. wt. $6x10^5$
Hemicellulose	Branched chain, contains pentoses/hexoses
Lignin	Major component of wood, adds stiffness
Pectins	Heteropolysaccharides from citrus fruit, apples
Gums, mucilages [a]	Attract water, thicken and become slippery
Algal polysaccharides [b]	From seaweed

[a] Karaya, tragacanth, guar, sterculia are examples.
[b] Agar and alginic acid are the principal components.

Particle size can influence the ability of fiber to retain water, and the intrinsic ability of the fiber to attact water also varies: per gram, bran can retain about 4.5 g water compared to 0.4 and 2 g water retained by potatoes and carrots, respectively (McConnell et al. 1974). The physical properties of fiber may be modified by bacterial action in the gut. Bile acids, which are normal components of the body, can bind to many types of fiber and contribute to its effects because they stimulate the movement of water into the lumen of the lower intestine (Binder 1977; Gaginella and Bass 1978; Nell and Rummel 1984).

Studies have revealed an association between large bowel cancer and high faecal bile acid concentrations in the presence of anaerobic bacteria capable of dehydrogenating the bile acid nucleus (Heaton 1972; Hill et al. 1975). The regulatory effects of fiber on colonic microbial metabolism, dilution of colonic contents, and adsorption of toxic materials (secondary bile acids like lithocholate) make it of potential value in the prevention of colon cancer (Cummings 1978).

There are a number of drug interactions that relate to the ability of fiber and hydrophilic colloids to bind or trap vitamins and other substances. Bile salts are bound by cellulose, which over the long term can reduce serum cholesterol levels. The absorption of the cardiac glycoside digitoxin and the antibiotic nitrofurantoin is said to be reduced by the synthetic hydrophilic laxative carboxymethylcellulose (Gullikson and Bass 1984).

Hydrophilic colloids become sticky and slippery in water, so they not only increase the fecal mass with resulting mechanical stimulation of the gut but they also soften the feces. Another mechanism that contributes to the laxative action of these substances is the formation of osmotically active metabolites by the intestinal bacterial flora (Ornstain and McLain Baird 1987). Hydrophilic colloids are useful in obese patients, as they also tend to cause a reduction in appetite. They are sometimes used in cases of diverticular diseases and hemorrhoids. In normal people the prolonged use of bran and hydrophilic colloids may cause luminal blockage (intestinal obstruction), especially if not taken with enough oral fluid (generous amounts of water should be prescribed with all bulk-forming laxatives).

5.5 Bran

Bran has been recognized as a laxative since 430 B.C., when Hippocrates is said to have stated that "whole meal bread clears out the gut and passes through an excrement, white bread is more nutritious; it makes less feces." (McCance and Widdowson 1955). The addition of bran to the diet softens the fecal consistency and increases transit through the intestinal tract. About 20 g bran daily is considered the minimum amount to produce a laxative effect. Bran is particularly useful in treating the spastic-type constipation associated with irritable bowel syndrome, although it can take several weeks before symptoms are relieved. The increased bulk produced by bran is also believed to be beneficial in diverticular disease of the colon (Hodgson 1972; Painter et al. 1972). Patients with atonic (or hypotonic) constipation may not be responsive to treatment with bran because of neuromuscular damage associated with chronic debility, old age or chronic laxative abuse.

By itself, bran is not very palatable. It is difficult to mix with water but can be consumed in the form of bran flakes or by adding it to baked goods or other foods. Many patients will experience bloating due to increased production of intestinal gas related to bacterial degradation of the components of bran. This symptom will usually disappear with time. It is important that adequate fluid intake be maintained for patients taking bran for constipation. Bran should not be employed in individuals with intestinal ulceration, stenosis or adhesions.

5.6 Psyllium (plantago)

The cleaned, dried, ripe seeds of *Plantago psyllium* Linne, or *P. indica* Linne, known in commerce as Spanish or French psyllium seed or of *Plantago ovata* Forskal, known in commerce as Blond psyllium or Indian plantago seed are the source of psyllium laxative. These plants, which are annual, caulescent and pubescent herbs, belong to the Plantaginaceae family; native to Asia and the Mediterranean countries, they are cultivated extensively in Europe (Spain), India and Pakistan. However, India is one of the main producers of this drug, which is cultivated in the State of Gujarat (Husain 1992). The seeds (Fig. 18) contain 10 to 30% of a substance which is hydrophilic and in water produces a mucilaginous mucoid-like substance. The mucilage absorbs water in the digestive tract which is also lubricates. It absorbs toxin and thus may be useful in dysentery as well as in diarrhea and constipation. Obviously, it is necessary to drink large amounts of water when taking this drug (Tyler

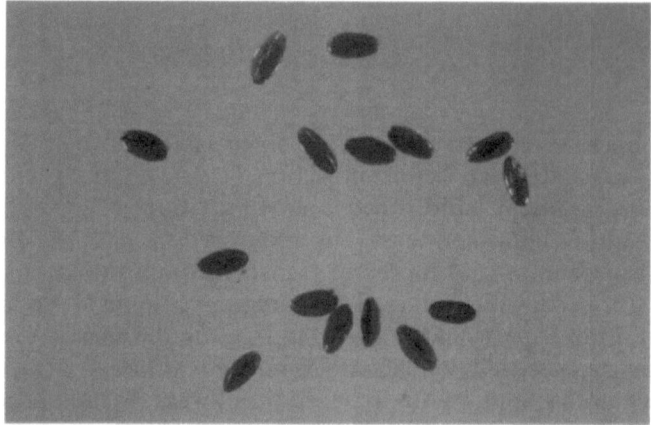

Fig. 18. Psyllium seeds

et al. 1988). It is used in amounts of 5-10 g (2 heaping teaspoonfuls) one to three times daily, usually suspended in juice, milk or water.

Psyllium is useful in treating spastic as well as atonic constipation, in the management of hemorrhoids and when excessive straining must be avoided following anorectal surgery. Although not associated with major drug interactions, psyllium is said to reduce serum cholesterol (if used long-term) by interference with reabsorption of bile acids (Forman et al. 1968). A relatively common side effect is an allergic reaction to psyllium. Sensitization (with asthmatic symptoms) after chronic inhalation of psyllium powder has been reported in atopic individuals (Brunton 1990). It may cause also renal pigmentation (if the seeds are ground or chewed).

Psyllium is combined with senna (Agiolax®) or chemicals such as anhydrous dextrose, sodium, bicarbonate, monobasic potassium phosphate, citric acid (Metamucil®).

In addition to its medicinal use, psyllium is also employed in chocolates, candies, ice-cream and corn flakes.

5.7 Alginic acid/Agar

The cell walls of certain brown algae of the species *Fucus* (*Fucus vesiculosus L.*), *Laminaria* and *Macrocystis* (*Macrocystis pyrifera L.*) which grow on the rocks along the north Atlantic coast, contain polysaccharides, such as alginic acid, that are hydrophilic. The principal component of alginic acid is a polyuric acid composed of D-mannuronic and L-guluronic residues. Alginic acid is a colorless and tasteless powder that forms a colloidal solution with a mucilaginous character. However large amounts are used as thickening agents in the alimentary industry (ice cream, chocolate, milk, salad dres-

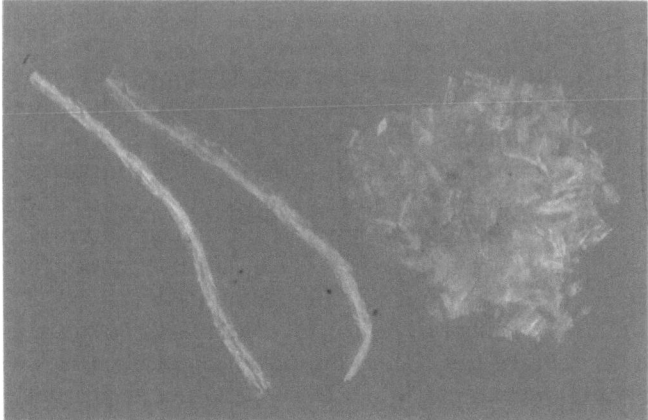

Fig. 19. Agar

sings, confectionary). Algin, the sodium salt of alginic acid, is also used for suspending cosmetic preparations and for other industrial purposes.

Agar is obtained from different species of algae, viz. *Gelidium*, *Gracilaria* and *Euchema*. These algae grow along the coasts of the United States, Spain, New Zealand, Australia, South Africa, and western South America. Agar occurs as bundles, consisting of thin, agglutinated strips (Fig. 19), or in granulated forms. It contains approximately 90% polysaccharides, comprised of agarose and agaropectin; the remaining 10% is water, nitrogen compounds and lipids. Agars from the different geographical sources have slightly different properties, but all agars swell in water and increase the moisture of the stool, thus producing a laxative effect. Sometimes it can take up to a week after initiating therapy with over 400 g agar before a benefit is realized.

5.8 Tragacanth

The dried, gummy exudate from *Astragalus gummifer* Labillardiere (family Fabaciae) or other Asiatic species of *Astragalus* provide the laxative tragacanth. Related products are karaya (sterculia) gum and bassora gum. The gums are collected in the period of March to June. After being dried and triturated they become a fine white powder with a slight smell of acetic acid. They contain a mucilaginous substance which can absorb up to 40 times its own volume of water. They also reduce the fermentative and putrefying processes. These gums are available in a variety of proprietary preparations and are used as bulk laxatives. Allergic reactions such as urticaria, rhinitis, atopic dermatitis, and asthma have been attributed to these agents.

5.9 Other fibers

There are other different vegetable substances which contain mucilaginous products that swell upon contact with water. These include the roots, leaves and flowers of altheae, the leaves and flowers of mallow, and the roots and flowers of viola. These vegetable substances may be used either alone (seldomly) or as adjuncts with other products for acute or chronic constipation. Their action is gentle and without side effects. The presence of tannins and saponins can reduce or increase the laxative action. They are thought to have a protective action on inflamed mucosa.

Malva silvestris (family Malvaceae) is an annual or biannual herbaceous plant found in central Europe and in the Balkan peninsula. The flowers (gathered before full flowering) and the leaves contain mucilaginous substances (galacturonic acid, galactose, methylpentose) and antocians. *Althaea officinalis* (family Malvaceae) is an annual herbaceous plant that grows in cool and humid parts of Europe and Asia. The roots (collected in autumn), the flowers that bloom from July to August, and leaves are used. About 30% of the plant material is mucilaginous substances composed of D-galacturonic acid and methylpentoses; 25% is starch. Other constituents are mineral salts, asparagine and betaine. *Viola odorata* (family Violaceae) is an herbaceous plant found on all the continents. The flowers, roots, leaves and seeds contain mucilaginous components and saponins. The roots also contain an alkaloid with emetic activity. It is believed that the saponin component acts on the mucosa. At the same time, the mucilage formed in the intestine has a soothing, emollient action that may contribute to its laxative effect.

5.10 Other laxative herbs and fruits

It should be noted that certain vegetables and fruits such as tamarind, cassia, blackberries, and dates may have a laxative action when consumed in sufficient quantities. This is due to their organic acid (citrate, tartrate) and sugar content. Tamarind pulp is obtained from the fruit of the *Tamarindus indica* Linne (family Cesalpinaceae), an evergreen tree found in India and tropical Africa (Fig. 20). The fruits are hanging pods, lumpy in relation to the seeds. The seeds are imbedded in a soft, yellowish substance (pulp) with a slightly acid taste and a particular odor. The pulp contains about 20% organic acid (tartaric, citric, malic) in the free form and as potassium salts, and about 20-30% mucilaginous substances and sugars. Tamarind laxative is taken in the form of jam or syrup. The dose is 40-60 g for adults and 1-2 g for children in cases of chronic constipation.

The pulp of cassia is obtained from the fruits of the *Cassia fistula* (family Leguminosae), a tree cultivated in tropical regions (Fig. 21). The fruits are

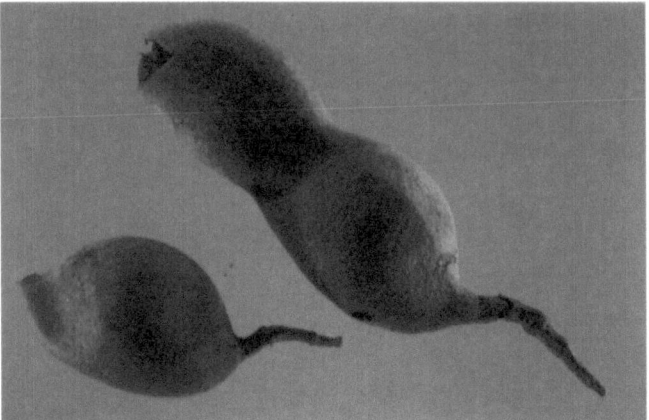

Fig. 20. Fruit of *Tamarindus indica*

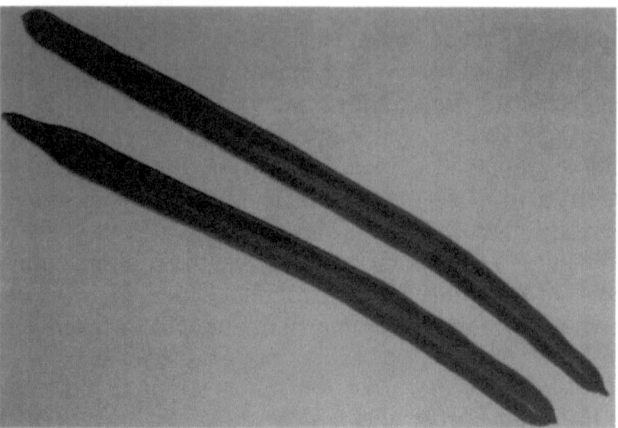

Fig. 21. Fruit of *Cassia fistula*

cylindrically shaped pods rounded at the extremities. The interior is divided into numerous sections filled with a blackish pulp which has a particular odor and sweetish taste. The pulp contains citric acid, tannic substances, pectin, anthraquinone derivatives (1%) and fructose (70%). It is used in the form of jam or syrup as a mild laxative for children. The dose is 40-60 g (3-5 g for every year of age).

Plums (*Prunus domestica*, Rosaceae) have an excellent laxative action at doses of 50-100 g. The laxative effect of plums is due to their content of fruit acid (2%), inverted sugar (50%) and oxyphenisatin (small amounts). Consuming soaked plums for breakfast enhances the action of a fiber-rich diet. Blackberries (*Rubus fruticosus*, Rosaceae) in the form of jam and syrup have a laxative action at doses of 40-80 g. Many other fruits, expecially if not very ripe, act as a laxative probably through a combined action of their fiber and osmotic effects of their natural sugars. The sugar content is 12% in figs, 25% in fresh grapes, 70% in raisins and 40% in plums.

6. Natural Laxatives of Mineral Origin

6.1 Inorganic salts

The action of saline laxatives lies in the presence of anions and cations which are poorly absorbed by the intestinal mucosa which behaves like a semipermeable membrane. The presence of these ions in the intestine leads to water retention in order to maintain an osmotic equilibrium, with indirect stimulation of peristalsis. The laxative action is related to the extent that the salts exert an osmotic effect, which can account for the greater laxative effect of some salt combinations compared to others (Table 9). Some salts reduce the pH in the colon and this may contribute to the laxative effect (Bennett and Eley 1976).

Table 9. Relative effectiveness of inorganic salts as osmotic laxatives

	Relative effect of equivalent dose
Anhydrous sodium sulfate	1.0
Crystalline sodium sulfate	1.4
Magnesium sulfate	1.5
Sodium phosphate	1.6
Sodium tartrate	2.0
Sodium citrate	2.3
Magnesium citrate	3.7

When saline laxatives are used, some of the salts are absorbed. This is relevant in patients with impaired renal function in whom hypermagnesemia has been observed (Kinnunen and Salokannel 1987). Saline laxatives are used orally or as an enema in preparation for radiological examinations, to expel parasites and in cases of poisoning. They are not advisable in cases of intestinal inflammation. Magnesium salts are contraindicated in patients with impaired renal function or congestive heart failure. Saline laxatives have the disadvantage of being bitter and of possibly causing damage to the intestinal mucosa (Bretagne et al. 1981; Meisel et al. 1977).

Magnesium sulfate ($MgSO_4$) is also known as English salt or Epson salt. The crystals are odorless with a bitter taste. They are taken orally, dissolved in water. The dose is 5-15 g. Magnesium sulfate may release cholecystokinin, a hormone that influences peristalsis and intestinal secretion and thus could be responsible for the laxative action (Harvey and Read 1973, 1975), although this theory is not well supported. Nitric oxide may be involved in the action of MgSO₄ (Izzo et al. 1994, 1996a).

Magnesium hydroxide is available in tablets; the usual dose is 2-4 g. An aqueous suspension of magnesium hydroxide (7.0-8.5%) is also available as a standard preparation (milk of magnesia); the usual dose is 15 mL. Other magnesium salts, i.e. carbonate, oxide, and phosphate, have similar laxative properties but are more commonly employed as gastric antacids.

Magnesium citrate is a pleasant tasting salt. The preparation magnesium citrate solution is a flavored solution containing the equivalent of 1.5-1.9 g magnesium oxide per 100 mL. Citric acid and sodium bicarbonate are added in excess to make the solution effervescent. The dose employed is 200 mL.

Sodium sulfate is also called Glauber salt and comes as a white hygroscopic, odorless powder with an unpleasant taste. The dose is 15 g for a cathartic effect and 3-6 g for a laxative effect.

Sodium phosphate comes in the form of transparent odorless crystals with a slightly alkaline taste. The dose is 4-8 g. Of all the saline purgatives it is the most palatable. A better tasting preparation, however, is effervescent sodium phosphate, a mixture of sodium phosphate, sodium bicarbonate and citric acid. The recommended dose is 10-20 g.

Sodium and potassium tartrate or La Rochelle salt forms colorless crystals with a bitter taste. It is slightly effervescent in dry air. The normal dose is 10 g. These salts when added to sodium bicarbonate and tartaric acid form an effervescent powder (Seidlitz powder). In practice tartaric acid is dissolved separately in water and mixed with the other two salts in equal parts just before use.

6.2 Mineral oil - A lubricant

It has been recognized early on in therapeutics that in certain instances defecation can be facilitated by the oral administration of various oily substances. These were originally classified as lubricants or emollients, and indeed this is probably an accurate description of how these oily substances act within the intestinal lumen. They are used especially after abdominal surgery or hemorrhoidectomy, or sometimes in pregnancy to reduce straining during defecation.

Mineral oil (liquid paraffin) is a purified mixture of hydrocarbons that is a colorless, transparent, odorless and virtually tasteless liquid. It is sometimes stabilized with 0.001% α-tocopherol. Usually the heavy form of the oil is employed as a laxative. The oil is believed to be virtually non-absorbable so that it remains in contact with the chyme and eventually the feces as they move from the small intestine through the colon. It is possible that some of the oil also coats the mucosal lining thus preventing (or retarding) fluid absorption. This would maintain moisture within the fecal mass. The normal dose of mineral oil is about 15 mL orally.

There are several undesirable effects of mineral oil when used as a laxative (Becker 1952). The most common of these is that the oil "leaks" from the body, causing rectal and anal irritation and itching (Jones and Gotting 1972), and may retard the healing of tissues after rectal or anal surgery. Because the oil can serve as a solvent or vehicle for lipid-soluble vitamins such as vitamins A, D, E and K (as well as lipid-soluble drugs), the absorption of these substances may be reduced. Thus, overuse can lead to deficiencies in the lipid-soluble vitamins. If this occurs on a chronic basis, the lack of vitamin D may promote osteoporosis especially in the elderly who would be prone to use this method of laxation; the lack of vitamin K may diminish the production of important blood clotting factors. Thus, episodes of bleeding and internal hemorrhaging may occur. Another potential problem, especially in infants and the elderly is lipoid pneumonia (Freiman et al. 1940), whereby lipid droplets enter the lungs after reflux from the stomach. For these reasons habitual use of mineral oil must be avoided.

7. Synthetic Laxatives

7.1 Diphenylmethanes

Also known as triarylmethane derivatives, this group of synthetic laxatives includes phenolphthalein, bisacodyl, picosulfate and oxyphenisatin. The later two drugs are not available in the United States but are used in Europe. All of these drugs decrease glucose and electrolyte absorption in the small intestine; they may also evoke active secretion of ions into the intestinal lumen (Farak et al. 1985; Ewe 1987; de Witte et al. 1991) and alter intestinal motility (Leng-Peschlow 1986) mostly in the colon (Forth et al. 1966). The mechanisms of action are unclear for all these drugs because of conflicting data from different experimental preparations. Some results indicate increases in prostaglandins and cyclic nucleotides (Rachmilewitz et al. 1980; Autore et al. 1984; Farak and Nell 1984; Capasso et al. 1986) or changes in mucosal permeability (Saunders et al. 1975, 1977; Meisel et al. 1977). Others show inhibition of Na^+, K^+-ATPase (Donowitz and Welsh 1987). Their effects on motility are inconsistent and poorly characterized (Gullikson and Bass 1984). These laxatives, like castor oil and the anthraquinones, probably act through causing multiple changes in normal gut physiology. They usually do not act in less than 6 h after oral administration; therefore they are taken at bedtime to produce their effect the next morning.

7.1.1 Phenolphthalein

This white, crystalline or amorphous tasteless and odorless powder was synthesized in the 1800s. Its laxative properties were discovered when it was added to wine in Hungary to increase the consistency and intensity of its color. The positioning of two *para*-hydroxyl functional groups on the phenyl rings of the molecule (Fig. 22) is similar to the orientation of the hydroxyl groups in the amphipathic (hydrophilic/lipophilic) dihydroxy bile acid molecules, which are secretagogues and laxatives (Phillips and Gaginella 1977; Binder 1977).

Phenolphthalein, like castor oil and the anthraquinones, is often classified as a stimulant or "contact" laxative but there is no evidence of a direct stimulating effect on intestinal motility in humans. Phenolphthalein acts mainly on the small intestine. It exerts an anti-absorptive/pro-secretory effect on electrolytes and water in the small intestine. This leads to fluid accumulation

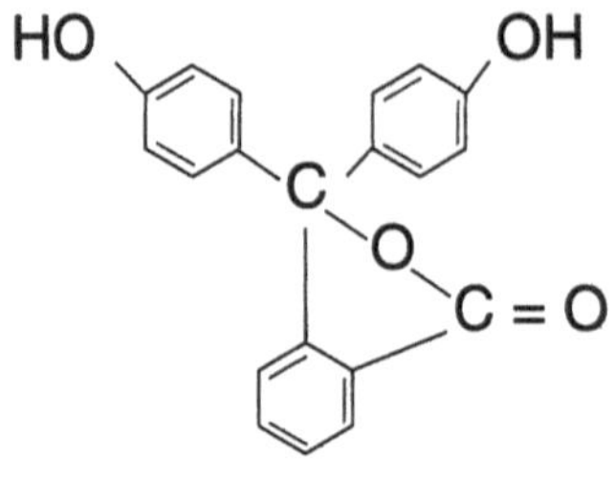

Fig. 22. Phenolphthalein

in the lumen, a less viscous stool and laxation. It is not entirely clear how phenolphthalein induces its effect on fluid transport, but it is believed to be partly through inhibition of active absorption of sodium across the basolateral membrane of the epithelial cells. Phenolphthalein also releases mucosal prostaglandin E (Buebler and Juan 1978) and causes exfoliation of small intestinal villus tips (Saunders et al. 1978), implying increased mucosal permeability and epithelial injury. These effects may be related to the recently reported effect of phenolphthalein in inducing the production of nitric oxide by the intestine (Gaginella et al. 1994). Nitric oxide is an intestinal secretagogue (Tamai and Gaginella 1993) which also relaxes intestinal smooth muscle; this leads to increased transit of lumenal contents through the bowel (*vide supra*, Chapter 4). However, changes in permeability and epithelial cell sloughing might also occur due to hydraulic flow of fluid from the interstitium into the lumen.

About 15% of the therapeutic dose of phenolphthalein is absorbed and the remainder is excreted in the feces. Once in the systemic circulation it is metabolized by the liver and cleared in the conjugated form (glucuronide) by the liver and kidney (Sund 1989). Of the amount absorbed, most of the phenolphthalein is excreted in the urine, where it may produce a pink color if the urine is alkaline. Some of the conjugated phenolphthalein is secreted back into the small intestine in the bile. This enterohepatic recycling of the drug probably contributes to its pharmacological effect. The glucuronide is poorly absorbed throughout the small intestine, thus delivering the conjugated drug to the lower ileum and colon where bacteria hydrolyze the glycosidic linkage and liberate the phenolphthalein. In this form it may act on the colonic mucosa (Forth et al. 1966) and possibly alter colonic neuromuscular function.

Phenolphthalein is relatively nontoxic but large doses can produce watery diarrhea and excessive loss of electrolytes in the stool. Allergic reactions have been reported (including Stevens-Johnson syndrome, lupus erythematosus and fixed-drug eruption), but these usually take the form of skin lesions which may persist for months. Deaths have been attributed to allergic reactions to phenolphthalein. Abuse of phenolphthalein can be discovered by alkalinizing the urine or feces: a red color indicates the presence of the drug. The usual oral dose is 60-100 mg (Munch and Calesnick 1960) and its action is seen in 6-8 h.

7.1.2 Bisacodyl

This diphenolic laxative (Fig. 23), used since 1953, was originally formulated for rectal administration, but now is also available as tablets for oral ingestion.

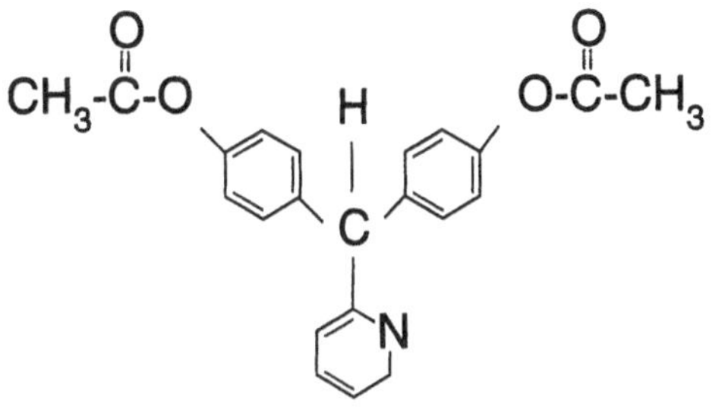

$$CH_3-\overset{\overset{O}{\|}}{C}-O \qquad\qquad O-\overset{\overset{O}{\|}}{C}-CH_3$$

Fig. 23. Bisacodyl

Only about 5% of an orally administered dose of bisacodyl is absorbed in humans. Some of the drug appears in the urine as the glucuronide. It is deacylated in the small intestine (Ferlemann and Vogt 1965), but both the native and deacylated forms of the drug are absorbed (Hillestad et al. 1982). These events may influence the absorption rate and extent of enterohepatic circulation of bisacodyl (Sund 1989).

After rectal administration in a suppository formulation, bisacodyl produces defecation in minutes, suggesting that the drug evokes a neural reflex upon contact with the rectal mucosa. The mechanism on the epithelium after

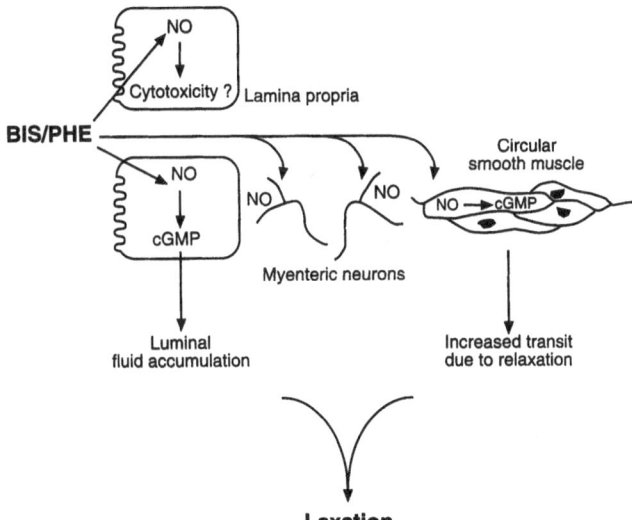

Fig. 24. Hypothetical nitric oxide (*NO*) involvement in laxative action of phenolphthalein (*PHE*) and bisacodyl (*BIS*). Reproduced with permission from Gaginella et al. (1994)

oral administration is complex, being partly due to inhibitory effects on Na$^+$, K$^+$-ATPase, release of prostaglandin E$_2$, stimulation of phosphodiesterase and adenylyl cyclase, and mucosal injury (Donowitz and Welsh 1987). Like phenolphthalein, nitric oxide appears somehow to be involved in the laxative effect (Gaginella et al. 1994). Figure 24 illustrates how nitric oxide may be involved in the mechanism of action of bisacodyl and phenolphthalein.

Bisacodyl tablets should be swallowed without chewing or crushing to avoid gastric irritation. They should be taken at least one hour prior to antacid in order to protect the enteric coating. Otherwise gastrointestinal upset and vomiting may occur. The laxative effect after oral ingestion occurs in 6-8 h. Mild proctitis and a burning sensation in the rectum have been reported after excessive (weeks) use of bisacodyl suppositories.

7.1.3 Picosulfate

Sodium picosulfate is a colorless, odorless, water soluble powder (Fig. 25). It is highly polar and poorly absorbed by the small intestine (Ferlemann and Vogt, 1965). As a consequence, picosulfate when ingested is conveyed to the large intestine, where it is hydrolyzed to its active diphenol (Sund 1989). Because it must reach the colon, its laxative action is usually not seen for 8-24 h.

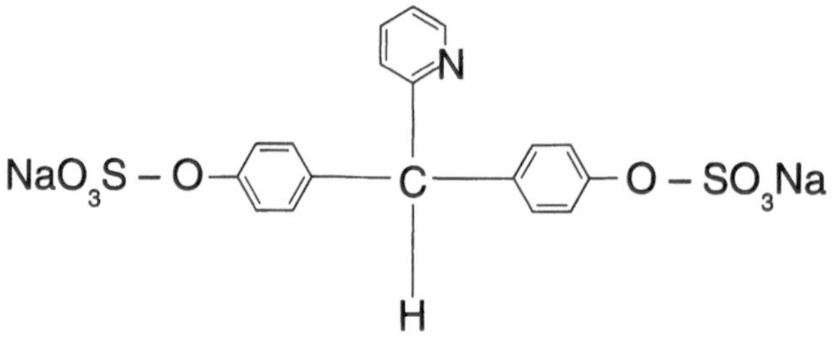

Fig. 25. Sodium picosulfate

7.1.4 Oxyphenisatin

This substance is present naturally in plums (Fig. 26). Its use is limited but it is included here mostly for historical reasons. It is poorly absorbable (Ferlemann and Vogt 1965) and it passes into the large intestine where it is hydrolyzed to its biologically active form (Moreto et al. 1979). However, due to liver toxicity (chronic hepatitis, cirrhosis) this drug has been removed from the market in many countries, but in other countries it is still obtainable in 5 mg suppository tablets. Its mechanism probably involves inhibition of Na$^+$, K$^+$-ATPase and increased permeability.

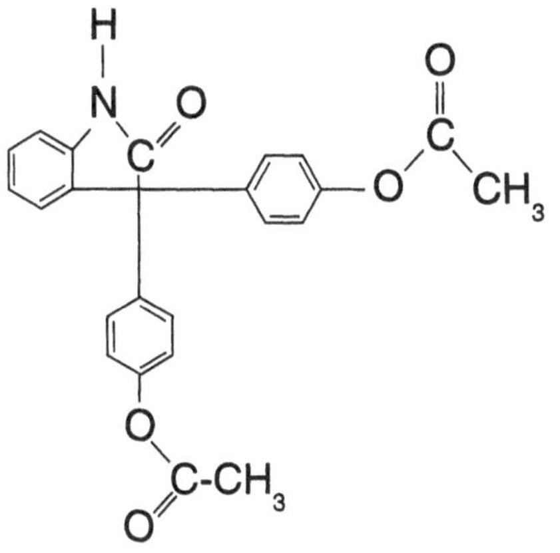

Fig. 26. Oxyphenisatin acetate

7.2 Dioctyl sodium sulfosuccinate

This drug is a surfactant (Fig. 27). Originally it was thought that dioctyl sodium sulfosuccinate (DSS) softened the stool by helping incorporate water through its wetting properties and emollient-like action. It is now known that DSS produces mucosal injury and epithelial cell toxicity (Saunders et al. 1975; Bretagne et al. 1981), which could explain its inhibitory effects on fluid absorption. DSS also inhibits Na^+, K^+-ATPase, but has inconsistent effects on cyclic AMP (Donowitz and Welsh 1987). It does not act as a lubricant of the mucosa.

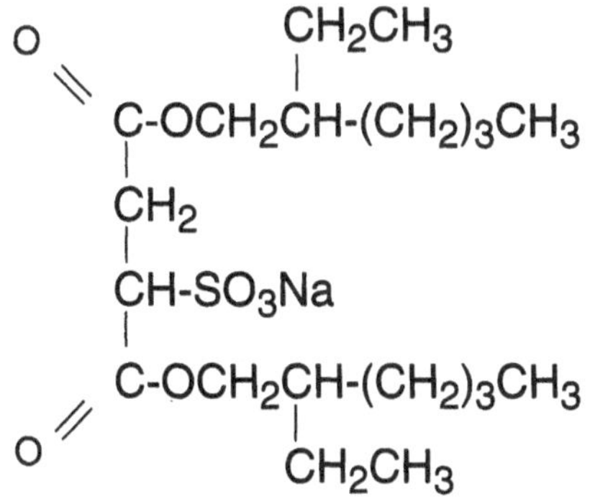

Fig. 27. Dioctyl sodium sulfosuccinate

   DSS is used whenever straining during a bowel movement must be avoided, as in postpartum women, and in patients with heart disease, with cardiovascular weakness or after anorectal surgery. Several products exist which combine DSS with anthraquinones or other laxatives. Hepatotoxicity has been reported when DSS was combined with oxyphenisatin, possibly because of its effects on mucosal permeability. DSS should not be given with a lubricant agent such as mineral oil, because absorption of the oil may produce systemic toxicity.

The usual dosage of DSS or its calcium containing form is 50-400 mg daily, as a single or divided dose. Oral solutions are also supplied containing 10 or 50 mg/mL. Usually 24-48 h are required for the laxative effect to be produced.

7.3 Sorbitol

Sorbitol is a polyalcohol (Fig. 28) with a sweet taste. It is poorly absorbed and thus exerts an osmotic effect throughout the small intestine. When ingested in amounts of 20-50 g it produces diarrhea. The sorbitol content of sugarless gum or mints (1.3-2.2 g per piece) is enough to produce a laxative effect in patients who consume 10 or more piece a day. Because of its ability to produce a pronounced laxative effect and its safety, sorbitol is often used in cases of drug poisoning.

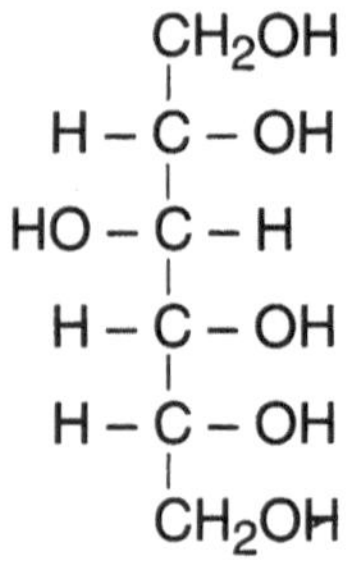

Fig. 28. Sorbitol

7.4 Lactulose

Lactulose consists of a disaccharide of galactose and fructose (Fig. 29). The small intestine lacks the disaccharidase to hydrolyze lactulose, therefore, it remains nearly unaltered and nonabsorbed until it reaches the colon. The bacteria metabolize it to lactic and acetic acids and carbon dioxide. Through

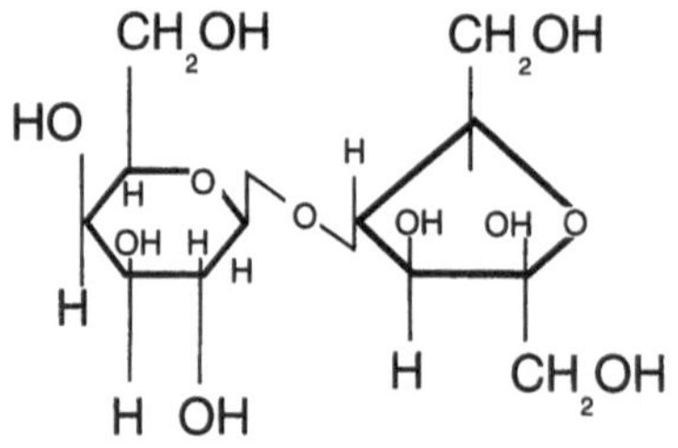

Fig. 29. Lactulose

direct mechanisms or alteration of colonic pH (a drop of colonic pH favors peristalsis), laxation is produced. A contribution from the osmotic activity of the unabsorbed lactulose in the small intestine is likely. Because lactulose is a bacterial nutrient, colonic bacterial mass increases with a consequential increase in fecal mass. Lactulose is a safe laxative even with chronic administration. Because lactulose reduces colonic pH and prevents the formation of co-carcinogenic secondary bile acids, it was postulated that it could prevent recurrence of colorectal adenomas as do antioxidant vitamins (Boisson 1990; Roncucci et al. 1993). Side effects of lactulose are abdominal discomfort and flatulence occuring in 20% of patients. Nausea and vomiting are not uncommon especially at high doses.

Lactulose is available as syrup. Laxation usually occurs in several days, with a dose of 15 mL (containing 10 g lactulose, comprised of 2.2 g of galactose, 1.2 g of lactose and 1.2 g of other sugars).

7.5 Methylcellulose

The methylether of cellulose, methylcellulose, is a granular or lumpy powder which is white or greyish-white, odorless and tasteless. When mixed with water it swells up to 25 times in volume. It is useful in maintaining flow in patients with colostomies, and in those with diverticular disease. It is used in adults at doses of 1-6 g per day; the pediatric dose is 500 mg 2-3 times daily. It is not absorbed in the digestive tract and does not interfere with the absorption of vitamins.

7.6 Polyethylene glycol

Polyethylene glycol (PEG) is an inert, water-soluble polymer that does not undergo either tissue or bacterial degradation (see Andorsky et al. 1990). It is absorbed from the intestinal tract in negligible amounts in normal subjects (< 0.06%) and in patients with inflammatory bowel disease (< 0.09%). The molecular weight of PEG can vary from about 200-8000. The high molecular weight form has been used at a concentration of 2-5 g/L as a marker of water absorption in intestinal perfusion studies in humans. More concentrated solutions of the high molecular weight form of PEG have been used orally (4 L over 2-4 h) to cleanse the bowel prior to endoscopy (Di Palma and Brady 1989). It has been suggested that because of its inert, non-absorbable and non toxic nature, PEG solutions may be useful for the safe treatment of chronic constipation (Andorsky et al. 1990). This treatment is not expected to impair normal motility and colonic function (i.e. "cathartic colon") when used long-term.

8. Laxative Abuse

Side effects have been described for the laxatives covered in this volume, and the potential for dependency on these drugs has also been described. Here we wish to comment on problems associated with prolonged use of these drugs. Indeed, over use (that is, continuous unwarranted use) of laxatives is *abuse* (Sarner 1976; Cummings 1974; Kacere et al. 1993).

The health practitioner must be suspicious of laxative abuse in a patient presenting with symptoms of weakness, aches and pains, diarrhea or an emotional disorder. There are remarkable descriptions in the literature of the behavior and the extent to which patients have gone to deceive their physician, nurse, pharmacist and family to gain sympathy for a disease from which they claim to suffer. Many of these individuals have unrecognized clinical problems, and they will not admit to taking laxatives. About 90% of confirmed laxative abusers are women (Thompson 1979). Patients that take any laxative in the recommended dose may complain of untoward effects like flatulence, cramping and abdominal pain (Shelton 1980). However, because constipation is often associated with abdominal complaints the causative role of the laxative is not always apparent.

Changes in muscular function, innervation and surface epithelium can occur at therapeutic doses when laxatives are over used (Meisel et al. 1977; Riemann et al. 1978). The anthraquinones are most commonly linked to neuromuscular changes which reduce the ability of the colon to transport fecal material, while castor oil and DSS are associated more with epithelial injury (Moriarty and Danson 1984; Muller-Lissner 1993). Bisacodyl and phosphate enemas induce superficial erosions, damage to the villi and disappearance of goblet cells (Meisel et al. 1977). Radiological examinations show a thinning of the intestinal wall, with disappearance of haustrations and dilatation of the

Table 10. Cathartic colon: morphological characteristics

Loss of haustration
Dilatation of intestinal lumen
Pseudostricture
Mucosa atrophy
Superficial ulcerations
Submucosal infiltrates (monocytes, eosinophils)
Mucosal and submucosal fibrosis

intestinal tract (Table 10). The intestine becomes hypomotile, with areas of prolonged spasm (pseudostrictures); there is smooth muscle atrophy with a decrease in wall thickness and damage to the myenteric plexuses. These changes are seen mostly in the ileum and colon, and represent cathartic colon (Tytgat and Mathus-Vliegen 1989) in the most serious instances (10% of cases). Morphological changes in the anus and rectum following long-term laxative use include cryptitis, anal fissures and strictures, perianal thrombosis and hemorrhoids. During the last 20 years not a single case of true cathartic colon has been described. The reason for this may be the absence in the marketplace of laxative preparations containing podophyllin, a poison of the metaphase of the cell cycle which induces sensorimotor neuropathy (Brunton 1990) and coma (Dobb and Edis 1984).

Nearly all the problems associated with laxative abuse are due to electrolyte

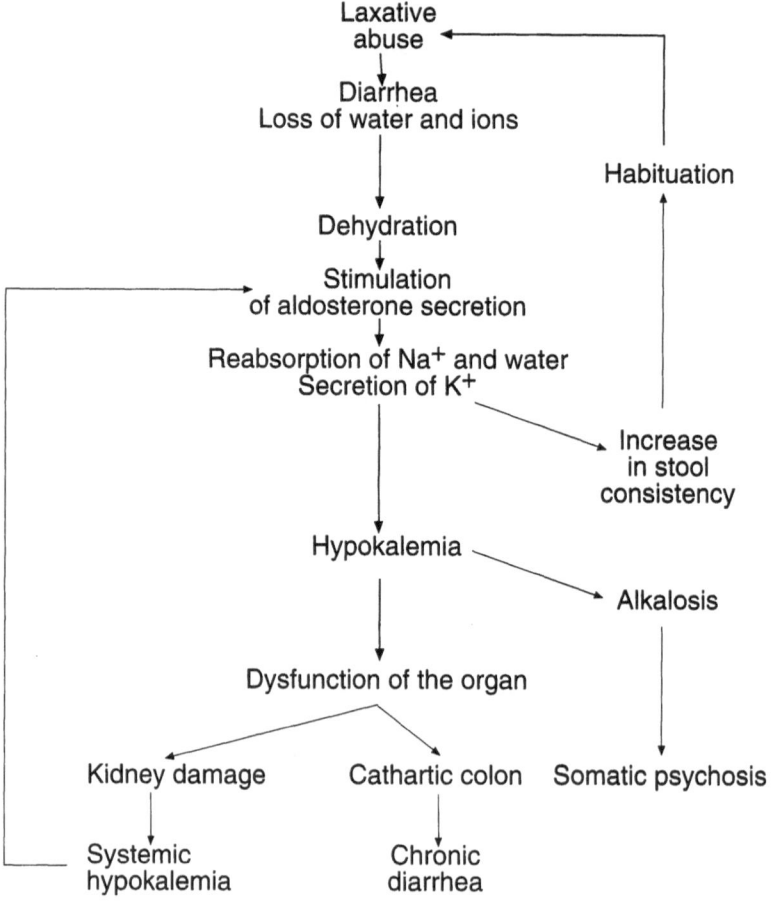

Fig. 30. Metabolic consequences of laxative abuse

imbalance (Fig. 30). The increased intestinal loss of K^+ can lead to hypokalemia while Na^+ loss can result in secondary hyperaldosteronism. This can exacerbate renal K^+ excretion leading to further reduction of colonic motility. This situation results in fatigue, muscular weakness, mental disturbances, steatorrhea, electrocardiographic abnormalities and kidney dysfunction (Schwartz and Relman 1953; Rawson 1966; Lemaitre et al. 1969; Dolman and Edmonds 1975; Fleming et al. 1975; Lesna et al. 1977; Osten et al. 1980; Levine et al. 1981).

8.1 Melanosis coli

Anthraquinone laxatives commonly produce *melanosis coli*, a deposition of lipofuscin-like pigment that gives the mucosa a mahogany to dark brown color. This is believed to be due to the sequestration of drugs by macrophages in the mucosa (Badiali et al. 1985), as illustrated in Fig. 31. Macroscopically, melanosis coli is limited to colorectal mucosa, but microscopically it can also be detected in the terminal ileum. The degree of coloration is most pronounced in the cecum and usually decreases toward the rectum (Koskela et al. 1989; Gobel, 1978). This condition, which may also occur in the absence of laxative abuse, was observed as early as 1830 and is seen with a prevalence of 4.7-8% in the normal population (Thompson 1979; Muller-Lissner 1993). Furthermore, ultrastructural studies have shown plication of the lateral cell membrane with widening of the intracellular space and granular inclusions within the colonocytes (Balasz 1986; Ghadially and Parry 1966).

Over 95% of 1,000 laxative abusers (most of whom took senna, cascara or aloe) were found at sigmoidoscopy to have melanosis (Cummings 1974; Steer and Colin-Jones 1975; Wittoesch et al. 1958; Spiessens 1991). In and of itself melanosis coli apparently does not have a deleterious effect on colon function, and it is usually reversible upon withdrawal of the laxative. In a case-controlled study, it was shown by the intake of senna-containing laxatives that melanosis coli could be generated in every patient during 4-13 months of treatment. Melanosis coli disappeared within 4-11 months after stopping the intake of senna drugs (Speare 1951). To detect abuse the feces can be screened chemically for the presence of anthraquinones (de Wolf et al. 1983).

Melanosis coli is considered a macroscopic and microscopic indicator of long-term use of anthranoid-containing laxatives. Because of the frequent administration of these laxatives it has been recently examined whether any relation might be detectable between consumption of laxatives, melanosi coli and development of colorectal cancer or adenoma in humans.

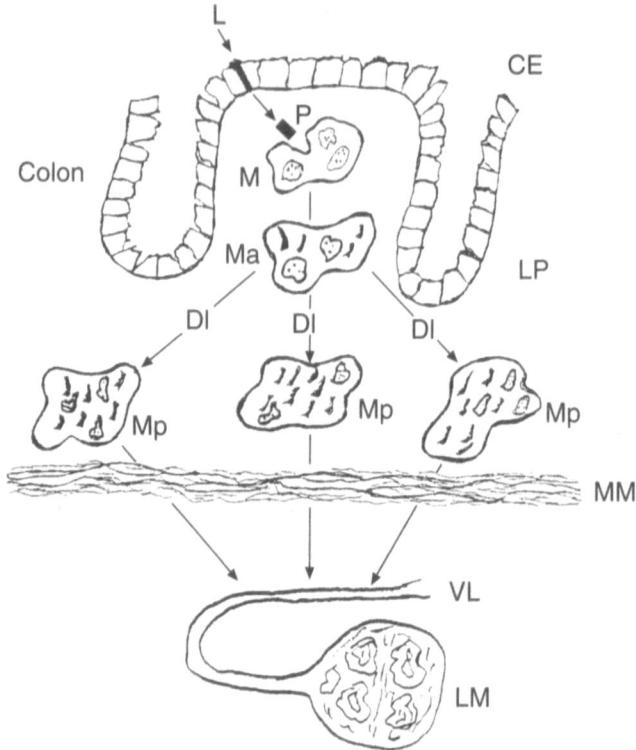

Fig. 31. Formation of melanosis coli in the mucosa of the colon or rectum. *L*, laxative; *P*, cellular fragment; *M*, macrophage; *Ma*, macrophage with apoptotic bodies; *Mp*, pigmented macrophage; *Dl*, lysosomal digestion; *VL*, lymphatic vessel; *LM*, mesenteric lymphnode; *CE*, epithelial cell; *LP*, lamina propria; *MM*, muscularis mucosae. The etiology of pseudomelanosis is still unclear. Laxatives could interact with colonic epithelial cells and induce migration of fragments of these cells into the spaces among the crypts. These cellular fragments would be phagosized by macrophages, and converted to lipofuscin-like pigments by enzymes present in lysosomes of the macrophages. As a consequence, the epithelium takes on a brown pigmentation. This is reversible upon removing the laxative because the macrophages with pigmentation will migrate towards the lymph nodes

8.2 Laxatives and colon cancer

Epidemiologic studies have given no evidence for any association between laxative use and the development of colorectal cancer (Boyd and Doll 1954; Nakamura et al. 1984; Kune et al. 1988; Kune, 1993; Nusko et al. 1993). Adenomas occur in patients taking laxatives, and the incidence is greated in patients with melanosis coli (Siegers 1992, 1993; Nusko et al. 1993). The increased incidence of adenomas in patients with melanosis coli might be explained by the easier detection of these lesions during endoscopy, since adenomatous tissue is not pigmented and appears as a white spot in a dark surrounding. Thus, colorectal adenoma cannot be attributed *per se* to melanosis coli. Another study, however, shows a small but significant risk for colorectal cancer associated with constipation and use of laxatives (Sonnenberg and Muller 1993). This risk appears to reflect the confounding influence of dietary habits rather than the primary influence of colonic inertia. Recently, an excessively high cell proliferation in sigmoid colon after an oral administration of sennosides has been demonstrated by Kleibeuker et al. (1995). These studies provide anecdotal evidence of an association between sennoside abuse and colon cancer. Although studies in rats suggest this possibility (Geboes et al. 1993; Toyoda et al. 1994), others did not show an increase in rectal epithelial cell proliferation after oral sennosides (Fireman et al. 1989). In addition, dietary exposure to high doses of senna or cascara glycosides for about 3 months did not cause the appearence of aberrant crypt foci (ACF) nor did it increase the incidence of ACF induced by 1,2-dimethylhydrazine (Mereto et al. 1996).

Large doses of danthron (a non-glycosidic synthetic anthraquinone which, in contrast to sennosides, passes into the blood stream in considerable amounts) and 1-hydroxyanthraquinone (a non-laxative metabolite of alizarin, one of the main constituents of *Rubia tinctorum* (Kawai et al. 1986)) have been demonstrated to cause adenomatous hyperplasia of the cecum and colon and to induce hepatocellular carcinomas in mice (Mori et al. 1986) and rats (Mori et al. 1985, 1990). An association has been suggested between danthron exposure (five years) and human cancer (leiomyosarcoma of the small intestine) in a 18-year-old girl (for ref. see Siegers 1992). However both danthron and *R. tinctorum* have not been used as laxative drugs for several years.

Mutagenic effects of anthraquinone derivatives have been shown *in vitro* (Brown and Brown 1976; Tikkanen et al. 1983; Mori et al. 1985; Westendorf et al. 1990; Muller et al. 1996), but the clinical relevance of these experimental results is still not clear. On the other hand it has been shown recently that an ethanol extract of Senokot (standardized senna concentrate) tablets is not mutagenic; to the contrary, it inhibits the mutagenicity of aflatoxin B_1 and other toxic substances, suggesting that an antimutagenic principle (s) is (are) present in the complex plant material (al-Dakan et al. 1995). The antimutagenic effect of Senokot extract could largely be due to an interaction with the metabolic activation of procarcinogens. The cytochemical effects of sennosides and other laxatives (bisacodyl, picosulfate) on rat colonic epithelial cells have been also studied recently (Yang et al. 1993). Consistent changes in acidic mucins, lectin soybean agglutinin and cytokeratin E_1 have been found in rats treated with anthranoid and non-anthranoid laxatives. However, there is no evidence that these changes lead to tumors in this rodent model. Similarly, Lyden-Sokolowski et al. (1993) found no carcinogenic potential of a senna extract given to rats over a period of 2 years. Therefore the cytochemical effects reported by Yang et al. (1993) are thought to be of functional origin and do not represent early precancerous lesions.

More recently Brusick and Mengs (1997) have submitted senna products and other anthraquinone compounds (emodin, aloe-emodin) to a large number of genetic tests. Assessment of the genotoxicity profile of these substances, in the light of kinetics studies, human clinical trials and rodent carcinogenicity studies, do not support concerns that senna pose a geno-toxic risk to humans when used periodically at therapeutic doses.

In conclusion, a carcinogenic risk from anthranoid laxatives in humans is based on evidence for a genotoxic potential of some anthranoids (danth-ron) and on *in vivo* carcinogenicity studies in animals. Clinical epidemio-logical studies (and experimental data) do not confirm this risk for anth-ranoid laxatives widely used (senna, cascara, rhubarb, aloe).

8.3 Neuronal injury

Damage to the autonomic nervous system of the colon has been reported after long-term use of anthraquinone and diphenylmethane laxatives (Smith 1968, 1973; Riemann et al. 1980). The functional significance of this dama-ge is unknown but it is possible that it represents injury to myenteric neu-rons that control colonic propulsive motility. In addition, activity or abnor-mal reactivity of these neurons might require the continued use of laxati-ves to maintain normal bowel function. However, laxative-induced dama-ge to the autonomic nervous system is poorly documented by experiments carried out both in laboratory animals and in patients; studies are restric-ted to silver staining of nerve fibers (Smith 1969; Dufour and Gendre 1984, 1988; Rudolph and Mengs 1988; Kierman and Heinicke 1989). These and other studies in patients (Smith 1973; Krishnamurthy et al. 1985; Kluck et al. 1987) do not allow a final conclusion. It is difficult to understand whether the abnor-malities observed in humans are a consequence of laxative intake or whether they represent pre-existing changes of unknown etiology which lead to a functional impairment (disordered absorption or motility). Furthermore, experimental studies show that chronic treatment with sennosides has no effect on spontaneous contractile activity of the rat colon *in vitro* (Odenthal and Ziegler 1988) and does not cause damage to the colonic nerve plexuses nor immunochemical changes (Dufour and Gendre 1984; Rudolph and Mengs 1988).

8.4 Habituation

Long-term abuse (or long-term therapeutic use) of laxatives is usually thought to result in habituation, i.e. the reduction or even disappearance of laxative response. However, this general assumption has not been properly demonstrated in patients (Leng-Peschlow 1992). Clinical studies do not show a loss of effect to laxatives (Muller-Lissner 1993). There are only occasional patients with a slow-transit constipation who report a need to increase the laxative dosage in order to maintain the desired effect. Habituation could be induced by damage to the organs involved in laxation (Leng-Peschlow and Mengs 1995) or by an increase of serum aldosterone levels. Since aldosterone increases sodium absorption and water reabsorption in the colon, the secretory effect of laxatives could be particularly reduced or abolished (Fleischer et al. 1969; Beubler 1985; Wanitschke 1987; Spiessens et al. 1991).

Studies carried out in rats also suggest that long-term sennoside treatment in diarrheagenic doses does not induce habituation in the sense of a reduced laxative effect and does not lead to secondary hyperaldosteronism (Leng-Peschlow et al. 1993).

After a thorough evacuation of the bowel by a senna preparation, several days are needed before a normal bowel movement can occur again. Thus, in the interim, a patient may become persuaded of being constipated and could be led to take a higher (or a daily) dose of laxative to receive a benefit (Capasso 1993), but this does not represent habituation. In fact, several investigations show that senna, when used sensibly, restores normal bowel function (Lowy 1960; Smith and Evans 1961; Haward and Hughes-Roberts 1962; Campbell-Mackie 1963).

Phenolphthalein is another frequently abused laxative. Excessive intake of this laxative can produce melanosis coli, electrolyte depletion, hyperaldosteronism, acid-base disturbances, malabsorption of glucose, protein and other nutrients, and possibly kidney damage. There is also the likelihood of dependency on continued use for normal bowel function. Habituation has not been proved however, for phenolphthalein. It is relatively simple to detect if a patient is abusing phenolphthalein merely by alkalinizing the stool or the urine and noting a pink color.

9. Methods Used to Study Laxative Drugs

Laxatives are generally studied with techniques which utilize the whole animal (*in vivo*). However, suitably prepared isolated systems (*in vitro*) may help to understand some aspects of the laxative action. The animals used for these studies are generally rats, mice, guinea pigs and rabbits. The simplest *in vivo* test consists of isolating the animals in individual cages and observing the percent of animals who have liquid or solid feces 8 hours after a particular treatment. Statistical comparison of the mean values of total diarrheal episodes in control (animals receiving a suitable vehicle) and test groups is made, and the results can be expressed graphically (Fig. 32). Since the examination of feces (i.e. to distinguish between soft, semi-solid and solid feces) is subjective it is preferable that the person who carries out the inspection is different from the one who administers the drugs.

Another test involves measuring the transit of a charcoal meal, which is easily visible, from the pylorus through the intestinal tract of mice or rats. Animals are fasted for 24 h prior to the experiments, pretreated with the test drug and 30 min later given orally the charcoal meal (0.2 ml of an aqueous suspension of charcoal in 5% arabic gum). The animals are killed by enflurane inhalation 20 min after the meal and the intestine and stomach are removed. The mean distance travelled by the charcoal is measured and compared with the control group. Results are expressed as the percentage of the total length of intestine. Radioactive markers such as [51]Chromium can also be used to measure transit through the intestine. An increase in propulsion rate indicates a laxative effect. The intestinal transit test is suitable for the study of laxatives which improve intestinal peristalsis. The test is not always appropriate also because some of the indicators have their own transit time which depends on, among other things, the consistency of the chewed food. To establish the site of action of laxatives, radio-opaque substances (bismuth carbonate and barium sulfate) are most useful; these allow a radiological examination of the transit of the fecal mass.

There are techniques which allow one to record the intestinal movement; others enable assessment of variations in the absorption and secretion of the colon or small intestine. A study of this type, the enteropooling test, simply consists of measuring the volume of intraluminal liquid of an isolated intestinal loop after having given the laxative to the animal. In this kind of study as with other techniques, the choice of anesthetic used is most important: it should not influence peristalsis or intestinal secretion.

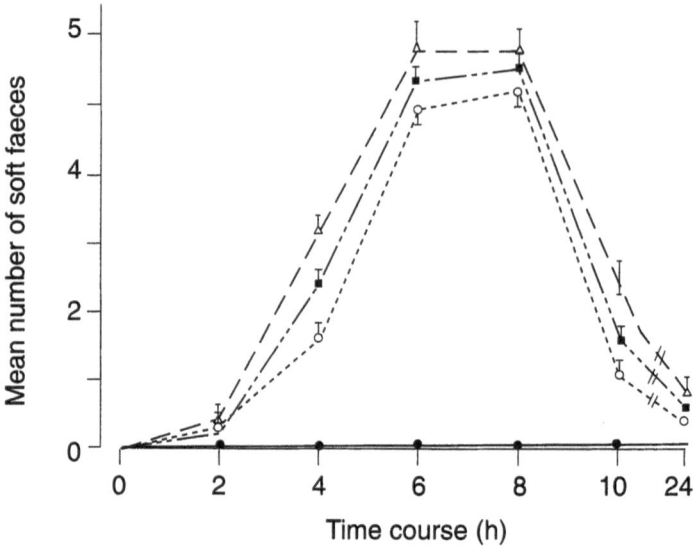

Fig. 32. Time course of the excretion of soft feces following oral treatment with senna in the following doses: ● 0; ○ 30; ■ 60; ▵ 90 mg kg^{-1}. Each point represents the mean ± s.e. of 10-12 rats. (From Mascolo et al. 1988)

Other tools useful to study laxatives are the Ussing chamber, isolated intestinal epithelia and isolated perfused intestinal segments. The Ussing chamber technique has proved useful in the study of electrolyte transport across many types of membranes. Several workers have modified the original apparatus proposed by Ussing and Zehran (1951), mainly altering the volume of the chambers or the surface area of membrane exposed to the bathing medium. Ion fluxes across both isolated rabbit ileum (Schultz and Zalusky 1964) and human intestine (Corbett et al. 1977) have been studied in this way. A modified Ussing chamber has been used to study the metabolism of phenolphthalein and other drugs in the animal intestine (Sund and Lauterbach 1986, 1987). The simplicity of the Ussing chamber technique makes it an attractive *in vitro* model system for the study of intestinal transport. However, as with all *in vitro* methods, there are limitations to the Ussing chamber technique, mainly arising from the absence of an intact mesenteric blood supply.

Isolated intestinal epithelia from both the small and large intestines have been used to study the toxic effects of laxatives and other drugs (Dawson and Schwenk 1989). Although isolated tissues have the advantage of being easy to prepare, toxicological studies are sparse.

Isolated perfused intestinal segments are useful tools to study intestinal absorption and metabolism (Parsons 1968) and the production of endogenous substances (Autore et al. 1990a). The technique involves cannulation

Force transducer

Syringe

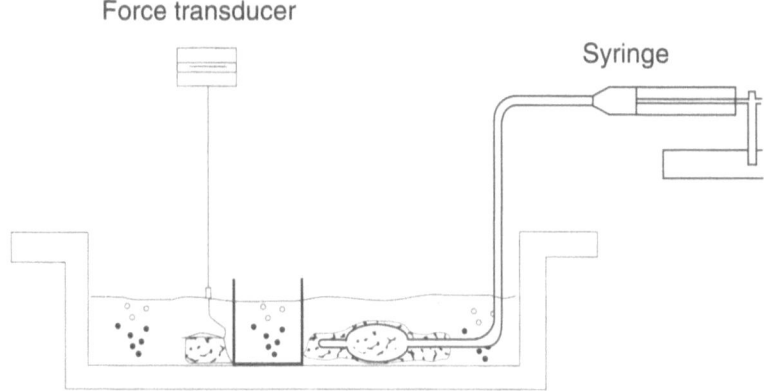

Fig. 33. Schematic drawing of experimental preparation for recording the reflex contraction of the circular muscle

of rat colon in situ. A soft polyethylene tube (about 3 mm outer diameter, 6 cm long) is inserted through a midline incision into the colon about 2 cm distal to the cecum, and the abdomen is closed. The animals are kept warm (23°C) with a heat lamp. The colon is flushed with an electrolyte (Tyrode's) solution until the effluent is clear. A second polyethylene tube is inserted about 3 cm into the rectum and the colon is perfused as above for 30 min before collecting small amounts (0.5-2 ml) of perfusate for analysis.

Tonini and Costa (1990) have developed a novel *in vitro* organ bath able to separate, by an intermediate compartment, the site of gut distension from the site of recording of the reflex contraction of the circular muscle (Fig. 33). By this experimental approach it is easy to ascertain the site of action of cholinergic receptor antagonists on the enteric excitatory reflex (EER) pathway and thus to establish the location of cholinergic and noncholinergic transmission along the reflex pathway of the EER in the intestine. This technique could be useful in the future to clarify the contribution of the different neurotransmitters in laxation.

Basic research studies are important in defining the mechanism(s) of action of laxatives. Classical as well as state-of-the-art molecular techniques, if applied to research on laxatives, will further our understanding about these widely used drugs. The reader is referred elsewhere (Gaginella 1995b) for more detailed information on methods for studying gastrointestinal motility and secretion.

10. Conclusions

The perception of the need for a regular bowel habit remains one of the reasons for the use of laxatives. Other reasons, such as the intake of food with a low fiber content, together with the lack of physical exercise, also contribute to the use of laxatives. Laxatives are frequently used as routine medication for patients in hospitals and are the most frequently prescribed drugs in long-term care facilities. However, they are of little use in the treatment of constipation due to organic causes or drugs. Nevertheless, today the use of laxatives is still valid in medicine. In the case of acute constipation, in some cases of chronic constipation (in order to accustom the patient to regulating the bowels), and in cases of constipation caused by atonia of the intestinal musculature, preference is given to anthraquinone laxatives (cascara, senna) because they are well tolerated and have a mild action.

However, the use of laxatives is not restricted to the treatment of constipation. They are used in cases of drug and food poisoning and after the administration of anthelmintics, where saline purgatives are preferred. Laxatives are prescribed to heart patients suffering from hemorrhoids and to patients bed-ridden for a long time as it is preferable to soften the feces. Before radiological exams, anthraquinone or saline laxatives are used, while before and after intestinal surgery lubricant agents are recommended.

When used appropriately, laxatives are extremely useful drugs. However in clinical medicine their excessive use can lead to abuse. The abuse of laxatives may cause loss of water, electrolytes and vitamin K. In more serious cases there can be ileal paralysis, renal lesions, oral malabsorption and habituation. In addition, when a single dose is too high, symptoms like abdominal pain, flatulence, bloating and diarrhea can correspondingly increase. All laxatives are contraindicated in patients with gastrointestinal disturbances, (cramps, colic, nausea, vomiting), with symptoms of appendicitis or with any undiagnosed abdominal pain.

Chronic constipation regardless of dietary factors (low fiber and high fat intake) or anthranoid exposure, does not increase the risk for colorectal cancer in humans.

11. References

al-Dakan AA, al-Tuffail M, Hannan MA (1995) Cassia senna inhibits mutagenic activities of benzo [α]-pyrene, aflatoxin B1, shamma and methyl methansulfonate. Pharmacol Toxicol 77: 288-292

Anderson AS (1986) Dietary factors in the etiology and treatment of constipation during pregnancy. Br J Obstet Gynaecol 93: 245-249

Andorsky RI, Major MD, Goldner F (1990) Colonic lavage solution (polyethylene glycol electrolyte lavage solution) as a treatment for chronic constipation: a double-blind, placebo-controlled study. Am J Gastroenterol 85: 261-265

Autore G, Capasso F, Mascolo N (1984) Phenolphthalein stimulates the formation of histamine, 5-hydroxytryptamine and prostaglandin-like material by rat jejunum, ileum and colon. Br J Pharmacol 81: 347-349

Autore G, Caliendo G, Pepe A, Capasso F (1990a) Perfusion of rat colon with sennosides, rhein and rheinanthrone. Dose related histamine release. Eur J Pharmacol 191: 97-99

Autore G, Calignano A, Mascolo N, Capasso F (1990b) Role of kinins in the laxation induced by castor oil. Pharmacol Life Sci Adv 9: 51-54

Badiali D, Marcheggiano A, Pallone S, Paoluzi T, Rausano G, Jannoni C, Materia E, Anzini S, Corazziari E (1985) Melanosis of the rectum in patients with chronic constipation. Dis Colon Rectum 28: 241-245

Balaa MA, Powell DW (1986) Prostaglandin synthesis by enterocyte microsomes of rabbit small intestine. Prostaglandins 31: 609-624

Balasz M (1986) Melanosis coli. Ultrastructural study of 45 patients. Dis Colon Rectum 29: 839-844

Baldwin WF (1963) Clinical study of senna administration to nursing mothers. Assessment of effects on infants bowel habits. Can Med Assoc J 89: 566-568

Bardon T, Deragnauncourt J (1985) Effects of platelet activating factor (PAF) on the digestive mobility in the conscious rat. Dig Dis Sci 30: 738-765

Bauer H (1977) Behandlung der Obstipation mit Laxantien in der gynakologischen Praxis. Ther Gegenwart 116: 2305-2312

Beck H, Beck K (1982) Schaufenster (Suppl Deutsche Apotheker Zeitung) 31: 33-34

Becker GL (1952) The case against mineral oil. Am J Dig Dis 19: 344-348

Bennett A (1992) Control of gastrointestinal motility. In: Capasso F, Mascolo N (eds) Natural drugs and the digestive tract. EMSI, Rome, pp 1-5

Bennett A, Eley KG (1976) Intestinal pH and propulsion: an explanation of diarrhea in lactose deficiency and laxation by lactulose. J Pharm Pharmacol 28: 192-195

Bennett PN (1988) Drugs and human lactation. Elsevier, New York, NY

Bennett WG, Cerda JJ (1996) Dietary fibers: Fact and fiction. Dig Dis 14: 43-58

Benveniste J (1988) PAF-acether, an other phospholipid with biological activity. In: Karnovsky ML, Leaf A, Bolis LC (eds) Biological membranes. Liss, New York, pp 73-85

Berridge M (1983) Phosphatidylinositol hydrolysis: a general transducing mechanism of calcium-mobilizing receptors. In: Turnberg LA (ed) Intestinal secretion. Knapp Drewett and Sons, Great Britain, pp 28-34

Beubler E (1985) Influence of chronic bisacodyl treatment on the effect of acute bisacodyl on water and electrolyte transport in the rat colon. J Pharm Pharmacol 37: 131-133

Beubler E, Juan N (1978) PGE-mediated laxative effect of diphenolic laxatives. Naunyn Schmiedeberg's Arch Pharmacol 305: 241-246

Beubler E, Juan N (1979) Effect of ricinoleic acid and other laxatives on net water flux and prostaglandin E release by the rat colon. J Pharm Pharmacol 31: 681-685

Beubler E, Kollar G (1985) Stimulation of PGE2 synthesis and water and electrolyte secretion by senna anthraquinones is inhibited by indomethacin. J Pharm Pharmacol 32: 248-251

Binder HJ (1989) Absorption and secretion of water and electrolytes by small and large intestine. In: Sleisenger MH, Fordtran JS (eds) Gastrointestinal disease, 4th ed. Saunders, Philadelphia, pp 1022-1045

Binder HJ (1977) Pharmacology of laxatives. Annu Rev Pharmacol Toxicol 17: 355-367

Binder HJ (1988) Use of laxatives in clinical medicine. Pharmacology 36 (Suppl 1): 226-229

Boisson J (1990) Essai du Duphalac (lactulose) pour le sevrage de laxatifs irritants. Le Concours Medical 10: 112-132

Bolton J, Field M (1977) Ca ionophore stimulated ion secretion in rabbit ileal mucosa: relations to actions of cyclic 3',5'-AMP and carbamylcholine. J Membr Biol 35: 159-163

Boyd JT, Doll R (1954) Gastro-intestinal cancer and the use of liquid paraffin. Br J Cancer 8: 231-237

Bretagne J, Vidon N, L'Hirondel C, Bernier JJ (1981) Increased cell loss in the human jejunum induced by laxatives (ricinoleic acid, dioctyl sodium sulphosuccinate, magnesium sulphate, bile salts). Gut 22: 264-269

Brooks SJH (1993) Neuronal nitric oxide in the gut. J Gastroenterol Hepatol 8: 590-593

Brown JP, Brown RJ (1976) Mutagenesis by 9,10 anthraquinone derivatives and related compounds in Salmonella thyphimurium. Mutat Res 40: 203-224

Brunton LL (1990) Agents affecting gastrointestinal water flux motility, digestants and bile acids. In: Goodman Gilman A, Rall TW, Nies AS, Taylor P (eds) The pharmacological basis of therapeutics, 8th edn. Pergamon Press, New York, pp 914-932

Brusick D, Mengs U (1997) Assessment of the genotoxic risk from laxative senna products. Environ Mol Mutagen 29: 1-9

Buckley TL, Hoult JRS (1989) Platelet activating factor is a potent colonic secretagogue with actions independent of specific PAF receptors. Eur J Pharmacol 163: 273-283

Bueno L, Frexinos J, Fioramonti J (1988) Role of motility in pathogenesis of constipation and diarrhea. Pharmacology 36 (Suppl 1): 15-22

Burgess DE (1972) Constipation in obstetrics. In: Jones FA, Godding EW (eds) Management of constipation. Blackwell Scientific, Oxford, pp 176-188

Cameron BD, Phillips MWA, Fenerty CA (1988) Milk transfer of rhein in the rhesus monkey. Pharmacology 36 (Suppl 1): 221-225

Campbell CM, Detwiller AK (1930) The lazy colon. Newer methods and latest advances of science in the treatment of constipation, 7th edn. The Educational Press, New York, p 312

Campbell-Mackie M (1963) The re-educative treatment of bowel dysfunction in infant and children. S Afr Med J 37: 675-678

Capasso F (1993) Lassativi e purganti. Aboca, Sansepolcro, pp 21 and 104

Capasso F, Tavares IA, Tsang R, Bennett A (1985) The role of calcium on eicosanoid production induced by ricinoleic acid or the calcium ionophore A23187. Prostaglandins 30: 119-124

Capasso F, Mascolo N, Autore G, Romano V (1986) Laxatives and the production of autacoids by rat colon. J Pharm Pharmacol 38: 627-629

Capasso F, Tavares IA, Bennett A (1992) PAF formation by human gastrointestinal mucosa/submucosa in vitro: release by ricinoleic acid and inhibition by 5-aminosalicylic acid. J Pharm Pharmacol 44: 771-772

Capasso F, Izzo AA, Mascolo N, Autore G, Di Carlo G (1993) Effect of senna is not mediated by platelet-activating factor. Pharmacology 47 (Suppl 1): 58-63

Capasso F, Di Carlo R (1994) Purganti, lassativi ed antidiarroici. In: Giotti A et al (eds) Farmacologia clinica e chemioterapia, 3ª ed, Vol 1. UTET, Torino, pp 1227-1231

Capasso F, Mascolo N, Izzo AA, Gaginella TS (1994) Dissociation of castor oil-induced diarrhea and intestinal mucosal injury in rat: effect of N^G-nitro-L-arginine methyl ester . Br J Pharmacol 113: 1127-1130

Caren JF, Meyer JH, Grossman MI (1974) Canine intestinal secretion during and after rapid distension of the small bowel. Am J Physiol 227: 183-188

Case RM, Hardcastle J, Hardcastle PT (1983) Calcium and secretory process. In: Turnberg LA (ed) Intestinal Secretion. Knapp Drewett and Sons, Great Britain, pp 24-28

Christensen J (1987) Motility of the colon. In: Johnson LR (ed) Physiology of the gastrointestinal tract, 2nd edn. Raven Press, New York, pp 665-693

Cline WS, Lorenzsonn V, Benz L, Bass P, Olsen WA (1979) The effects of sodium ricinoleate on small intestinal function and structure. J Clin Invest 58: 380-390

Code CF, Bass P, McClary GB Jr, Newnum RL, Orvin AL (1960) Absorption of water, sodium and potassium in small intestine of dogs. Am J Physiol 199: 281-288

Colombo P (1994) Trattamento della stipsi cronica in soggetti anziani. Arch Med Interna 46: 1-17

Corbett CL, Issacs PET, Riley AK, Turnberg LA (1977) Human intestinal transport in vitro. Gut 18: 136-140

Cummings JH (1974) Progress report: Laxative abuse. Gut 15: 758-766

Cummings JW (1978) Dietary fibre and colonic function. J R Soc Med 71: 81-86

Dawson JR, Schwenk M (1989) Isolated epithelial cells. Progress in Pharmacol Clin Pharmacol 7: 21-41

De Jonge HR (1975) The response of small intestine villous and crypt epithelium to cholera-toxin in rat and guinea-pig. Evidence against a specific role of the crypt cells in choleragen-induced secretion. Biochim Biophys Acta 381: 128

de Witte P, Dreessen M, Lemli J (1991) The influence of some anthracene and diphenylmethane derivatives on water and electrolyte movement in rat colon. Pharm Acta Helv 66: 70-73

De Wolf FA, Edelbrock PM, de Haas EJM, Vermeij P (1983) Experience with a screening method for laxative abuse. Hum Toxicol 2: 385-389

Di Palma JA, Brady CE (1989) Colon cleansing for diagnostic and surgical procedures: Polyethylene glycol-electrolyte lavage solution. Am J Gastroenterol 84: 1008-1016

Dobb GJ, Edis RH (1984) Coma and neuropathy after ingestion of herbal laxative containing podophyllin. Med J Aust 140: 495-496

Dolman D, Edmonds CJ (1975) The effect of aldosterone and the renin angiotensin system on sodium, potassium and chloride transport by proximal and distal rat colon in vivo. J Physiol (Lond) 250: 597-611

Donowitz M, Welsh MJ (1987) Regulation of mammalian small intestinal electrolyte secretion. In: Johnson LR (ed) Physiology of the gastrointestinal tract, 2nd edn. Raven Press, New York, pp 1351-1388

Douthwaith A, Goulding R (1957) Action of senna. Br Med J 4: 1414-1415

Dreessen M, Lemli J (1988) Studies in the field of drugs containing anthraquinone derivatives. The metabolism of cascarosides by intestinal bacteria. Pharm Acta Helv 63: 287-289

Dubecq JP, Palmade JL (1974) Etude de l'administration de Tamarine chez la mère qui allaite. Gaz Med Fr 81: 5173-5175

Dufour P, Gendre P (1984) Ultrastructure of mouse intestinal mucosa and changes observed after long-term anthraquinone administration. Gut 15: 1358-1363

Dufour P, Gendre P (1988) Long-term mucosal alterations by sennosides and related compounds. Pharmacology 36 (Suppl 1): 194-202

Duncan AS (1957) Standardized senna as a laxative in the puerperium. A clinical assessment. Br Med J 1: 439-441

Ewe K (1987) Effect of bisacodyl on intestinal electrolyte and water net transport and transit. Digestion 37: 247-253

Faber P, Strenge-Hesse A (1988) Relevance of rhein excretion into breast milk. Pharmacology 36 (Suppl 1): 212-220

Farack U, Nell G (1984) Mechanism of action of diphenolic laxatives: The role of adenylate cyclase and mucosal permeability. Digestion 30: 191-194

Farack U, Gruber E, Loeschke K (1985) The influence of bisacodyl on mucus secretion, mucus synthesis and electrolyte movements in the rat colon in vivo. Eur J Pharmacol 117: 215-222

Ferlemann G, Vogt W (1965) Entazetylierung und Resorption von phenolischen Laxantien. Arch Exp Path Pharmak 250: 479-487

Field M, Smith PL, Bolton JE (1980) Ion transport across the isolated small intestinal mucosa of the winter flounder *Pseudopleuronectes american*: II Effects of cyclic AMP. J Membr Biol 55: 157

Fingl E (1975) Laxatives and cathartics. In: Goodman LS, Gilman A (eds) The pharmacological basis of therapeutics, 5th edn. Macmillan, New York, pp 976-986

Fireman Z, Rozen P, Fine N, et al. (1989) Reproducibility studies and effects of bowel preparation on measurements of rectal epithelial proliferations. Cancer Lett 45: 59-64

Fleischer N, Brown H, Graham DY, Delena S (1969) Chronic laxative-induced hyperaldosteronism and hypokalemia stimulating Bartter's syndrome. Ann Intern Med 70: 791-798

Fleming BJ, Genuth SM, Gould AB, Kaminonkowski MD (1975) Effects of potassium and sodium replacement on the renin-angiotensin-aldosterone system. Ann Int Med 83: 60-62

Forman DT, Garvin JE, Forestner JE, Taylor CB (1968) Increased excretion of fecal bile acids by an oral hydrophilic colloid. Proc Soc Exp Biol Med 127: 1060-1063

Forth W, Rummel W, Baldauf J (1966) Wasser - und Elektrolytbewegung am Dünn - und Dickdarm unter dem Einfluss von Laxantien, ein Beitrag zur Klärung ihres Wirkungsmechanismus. Arch Pharmak Exp Path 254: 18-32

Freiman DG, Engelberg H, Merrit WH (1940) Oil aspiration pneumonia in adults: a study of 47 patients. Arch Intern Med 66: 11-38

Frexinos J, Staumont G, Fioramonti J, Bueno L (1989) Effects of sennosides on colonic myoelectrical activity in man. Dig Dis Sci 34: 214-219

Gaginella TS (1977) The management of gastrointestinal disorders. II. Use and misuse of laxatives. J Continuing Education of Pharmacy 1: 19-28

Gaginella TS (1990a) Eicosanoid-mediated intestinal secretion. In: Lebenthal E, Duffey M (eds) Secretory diarrhea. Raven Press, New York, pp 15-30

Gaginella TS (1990b) Receptor pharmacology of intestinal secretion. In: Lebenthal E, Duffey M (eds) Secretory diarrhea. Raven Press, New York, pp 163-178

Gaginella TS (1995a) Laxative drugs. In: Munson PL, Mueller RA and Breese GR (eds) Principles of Pharmacology. Chapman and Hall, New York

Gaginella TS (ed) (1995b) Handbook of methods in gastrointestinal pharmacology. CRC Press, Boca Raton

Gaginella TS, Bass P (1978) Laxatives: An uptade on mechanism of action. Life Sci 23: 1001-1010

Gaginella TS, Phillips SF (1975) Ricinoleic acid: current view of an ancient oil. Am J Dig Dis 20: 1171-1177

Gaginella TS, Hubel KA, O'Dorisio TM (1982) Vasoactive intestinal polypeptide and intestinal chloride secretion. In: Vasoactive intestinal polypeptide. Adv Peptide Hormone Res, vol 1. Raven Press, New York, pp 211-222

Gaginella TS, Mascolo N, Izzo AA, Autore G, Capasso F (1994) Nitric oxide as a mediator of bisacodyl and phenophthalein laxative action: induction of nitric oxide synthase. J Pharmacol Exp Ther 270: 1239-1245

Garcia-Villar R, Leng-Peschlow E, Ruckebusch Y (1980) Effect of anthraquinone derivatives on canine and rat intestinal motility. J Pharm Pharmacol 32: 323-329

Gattuso JM, Kamm MA (1994) Adverse effects of drugs used in the management of constipation and diarrhoea. Drug Saf 10: 47-65

Geboes K, Nijs G, Mengs U, Geboes KPJ, Van Damme A, de Witte P (1993) Effects of contact laxatives on intestinal and colonic epithelial cell proliferation. Pharmacology 47 (Suppl 1): 187-195

Ghadially FN, Parry EW (1966) An electro-microscope and histochemical study of melanosis coli. J Pharm Bact 92: 313-317

Gobel D (1978) Melanosis coli. Med Klin 73: 519-523

Grindlay D, Reynolds T (1986) The Aloe vera phenomenon: a review of the properties and modern uses of the leaf parenchyma gel. J Ethnopharmacology 16: 117-151

Gullikson GW, Bass P (1984) Mechanisms of action of laxative drugs. In: Csaky TZ (ed) Pharmacology of intestinal permeation II, vol 70. Springer-Verlag, Berlin Heidelberg New York, pp 419-459

Hattori M, Kim G, Motoike S, Kobashi K, Namba T (1982) Metabolism of sennosides by intestinal flora. Chem Pharm Bull (Tokyo) 30: 1338-1346

Hardcastle JD, Wilkins JL (1970) The action of sennosides and related compounds on human colon and rectum. Gut 11: 1038-1040

Harvey RE, Read AE (1973) Saline purgatives act by releasing cholecystokinin. Lancet 2: 185-187

Harvey RE, Read AE (1975) Mode of action of saline purgatives. Am Heart J 89: 810-812

Haubrich WS (1985) Constipation. In: Bockus (ed) Gastroenterology. Saunders, Philadelphia, pp 111-124

Haward LRC, Hughes-Roberts HE (1962) The treatment of constipation in mental hospitals. Gut 3: 85-90

Heaton KW (1972) Bile salts in health and disease. Churchill Livingstone, Edinburgh

Heiny BM (1976) Langzeitbehandlung mit einem pflanzlichen Laxativum. Serumelektrolyte und Säurenhaushalt. Arztliche Praxis 28: 563-564

Hill MJ, Drasar BS, Williams REO, Meade TW, Cox AG, Simpson JEP, Morson BC (1975) Faecal bile-acids and clostridia in patients with cancer of the large bowel. Lancet i: 535

Hietala P, Marvola M, Parviainen T, Lainonen H (1987) Laxative potency and acute toxicity of some anthraquinone derivatives, senna extracts and fractions of senna extracts. Pharmacol Toxicol 61: 153-156

Hillestad B, Sund RB, Buajordet M (1982) Intestinal handling of bisacodyl and picosulphate by everted sacs of the rat jejunum and stripped colon. Acta Pharmacol Toxicol 51: 388-394

Hodgson J (1972) Effect of methylcellulose on rectal and colonic pressure in treatment of diverticular disease. Br Med J 3: 729-731

Hormann HP, Korting HC (1994) Evidence for the efficacy and safety of topical herbal drugs in dermatology: part 1: anti-inflammatory agents. Phytomedicine 1: 161-171

Husain A (1992) Economic aspects of exploitation of medicinal plants. In: Akerele O, Heywood V, Synge H (eds) Conservation of Medicinal Plants. University Press, Cambridge, pp 125-140

Illingworth RS (1953) Abnormal substances excreted in human milk. Practitioner 171: 533-538

Ishii Y, Tanizawa H, Takino Y (1990) Studies of Aloe III. Mechanism of cathartic effect. Chem Pharm Bull 38: 197-200

Itasaka S, Shirataori K, Takahashi T, Ishikawa M, Kanedo K, Suzuki Y (1992) Stimulation of intramural secretory reflex by luminal distension pressure in rat distal colon. Am J Physiol 263: G108-G114

Izzo AA (1996) PAF and the digestive tract. A review. J Pharm Pharmacol 48: 1103-1111

Izzo AA, Mascolo N, Autore G, Di Carlo G, Capasso F (1993) Increased ex-vivo colonic generation of PAF induced by diphenylmethane stimulant laxatives in the rat, mice, guinea-pig and rabbits. J Pharm Pharmacol 45: 916-918

Izzo AA, Gaginella TS, Mascolo N Capasso F (1994) Nitric oxide as a mediator of the laxative action of magnesium sulphate. Br J Pharmacol 113: 228-232

Izzo AA, Gaginella TS, Capasso F (1996a) The osmotic and intrinsic mechanisms of the pharmacological laxative action of oral high doses of magnesium sulphate. Importance of the release of digestive polypeptides and nitric oxide. Magnes Res 9: 133-138

Izzo AA, Gaginella TS, Mascolo N, Borrelli F, Capasso F (1996b) N^G-Nitro-L-arginine methyl ester reduces senna- and cascara-induced diarrhoea and fluid secretion in the rat. Eur J Pharmacol 301: 137-142

Izzo AA, Sautebin L, Rombola L, Capasso F (1997) The role of constitutive and inducible nitric oxide synthase in senna- and cascara-induced diarrhoea in the rat. Eur J Pharmacol 323: 93-97

Jones FA, Gotting EW (1972) Management of constipation. Blackwell and Mott, Oxford

Kacere RD, Srivatsa SS, Tremaine WJ, Ebnet LE, Batts KP (1993) Chronic diarrhea due to surreptitious use of bisacodyl: case reports and methods for detection. Mayo Clin Proc 68: 355-357

Kantor JL, Cooper LF (1937) The dietetic treatment of constipation with special reference to food fiber. Ann Intern Med 10: 965-978

Kawai K, Mori H, Sugie S, Yoshimi N, Inoue T, Nakamura T, Nozawa Y, Matsushima T (1986) Genetoxicity in the hepatocyte/DNA repair test and toxicity to liver mitochondria of 1-hydroxyanthraquinone and several dihydroxyanthraquinones. Cell Biol Toxicol 4: 457-467

Kellogg JH (1921) The new dietetics. Modern Medicine Publishing, Battle Creek

Kierman JA, Heinicke EH (1989) Sennosides do not kill myenteric neurons in the colon of the rat or mouse. Neuroscience 30: 837-842

Kinnunen O, Salokannel J (1987) Constipation in elderly long-stay patients: its treatment by magnesium hydroxide and bulk laxative. Ann Clin Res 19: 321-323

Kinnunen O, Winblad I, Koistinen P, Salokannel J (1993) Safety and efficacy of a bulk laxative containing senna versus lactulose in the treatment of chronic constipation in geriatric patients. Pharmacology 47 (Suppl 1): 253-255

Kleibeuker JH, Cats A, Zwart N, Mulder NH, Hardonk MJ, de Vries EGE (1995) Excessively high cell proliferation in sigmoid colon after an oral purge with anthraquinone glycosides. J Natl Cancer Inst 87: 152-153

Kluck P, ten Kate FJW, Schouten WR, Bartels KCM, Tibboel D, van der Kamp AWM, Molenaar JC, van Blankenstein M (1987) Efficacy of antibody NF2F11 staining in the investigation of severe long-standing constipation. Gastroenterology 93: 872-875

Koskela E, Kulju T, Collan Y (1989) Prevalence, distribution and histologic feature in 200 consecutive autopsies at Kuopio University Central Hospital. Dis Colon Rectum 32: 235-239

Krishnamurthy S, Schuffler MD, Rohrmann CA, Pope CE (1985) Severe idiopathic constipation is associated with a distinctive abnormality of the colonic myenteric plexus. Gastroenterology 88: 26-34

Kune GA (1993) Laxative use not a risk for colorectal cancer. Data from the Melbourne colorectal cancer study. Z Gastroenterol 31: 140-143

Kune GA, Kune S, Field B, Watson LF (1988) The role of chronic constipation diarrhoea, and laxative use in the etiology of large bowel cancer. Data from the Melbourne colorectal cancer study. Dig Colon Rect 31: 507-512

Latven A, Sloane A, Munch J (1952) Biossay of cathartics. I. Emodine type. J Am Pharm Assoc 41: 548-552

Lawson M, Kern F, Everson GT (1985) Gastrointestinal transit time in human pregnancy: proliferation by postpartum normalization. Gastroenterology 89: 996-999

Lemaitre G, L'Herminé C, Decoulx M, Houlcke M, Linquette M (1969) Les lesions coliques par abus de laxatifs. Presse Med 77: 393-394

Leng-Peschlow E (1980) Inhibition of intestinal water and electrolyte absorption by senna derivatives in rats. J Pharm Pharmacol 32: 330-335

Leng-Peschlow E (1986) Acceleration of large intestine transit time in rats by sennosides and related compounds. J Pharm Pharmacol 38: 369-373

Leng-Peschlow E (1992) Senna and its rational use. Pharmacology 44 (Suppl 1): 1-52

Leng-Peschlow E, Mengs U (1995) Senna laxatives: safe and effective. Pharmaz Zeit 140: 668-674

Leng-Peschlow E, Odenthal KP, Voderholzer W, Muller-Lissner S (1993) Chronic sennoside treatment does not cause habituation and secondary hyperaldosteronism in rats. Pharmacology 47 (Suppl 1): 162-171

Lesna M, Hamlyn AN, Venables CW, Record CD (1977) Chronic laxative abuse associated with pancreatic islet cell hyperplasia. Gut 18: 1032-1035

Levine D, Goode AW, Wingate DL (1981) Purgative abuse associated with reversible cachexia, hypogammaglobulinaemia, and finger clubbing. Lancet 1: 919-920

Lium R, Florey HW (1939) The action of magnesium sulphate on the intestine of the cat. Quarterly J Exp Physiol 29: 303-319

Longo R (1980) Attività e metabolismo nel topo di componenti la corteccia di *Rhamnus frangula* e di prodotti sintetici a struttura antrachinonica. Boll Chim Farm 119: 669-684

Lowy A (1960) Bowel reabilitation in the chronically constipated patient. Int Rec Med 173: 303-305

Lyden-Sokolowski A, Nilsson A, Sjoberg P (1993) Two-year carcinogenicity study with sennosides in the rat: emphasis on gastrointestinal alterations. Pharmacology 47: 209-215

Maenz DD, Forsyth GW (1982) Ricinoleate and deoxycholate are calcium ionophore in jejunal brush borders. J Memb Biol 70: 125-133

Mahon R, Palmade J (1974) Traitement de la constipation chez la femme enceinte. Gaz Med Fr 81: 3259-3260

Mascolo N, Autore G, Izzo AA, Biondi A, Capasso F (1992) Effects of senna and its active compounds rhein and rheinanthrone on PAF formation by rat colon. J Pharm Pharmacol 44: 693-695

Mascolo N, Gaginella TS, Izzo AA, Di Carlo G, Capasso F (1994a) Nitric oxide involvement in sodium choleate-induced fluid secretion and diarrhoea in rats. Eur J Pharmacol 264: 21-26

Mascolo N, Izzo AA, Autore G, Barbato F, Capasso F (1994b) Nitric oxide and castor oil-induced diarrhea. J Pharmacol Exp Ther 268: 291-295

Mascolo N, Izzo AA, Barbato F, Capasso F (1993) Inhibitors of nitric oxide synthase prevent castor oil-induced diarrhoea in rats. Br J Pharmacol 108: 861-864

Mascolo N, Izzo AA, Gaginella TS, Capasso F (1996) Relationship between nitric oxide and platelet activating factor in castor oil-induced mucosal injury in the rat duodenum. Naunyn Schmiedebergs Arch Pharmacol 353: 680-684

Mascolo N, Meli R, Autore G, Capasso F (1988a) Senna still causes laxation in rats maintained on a diet deficient in essential fatty acids. J Pharm Pharmacol 40: 882-884

Mascolo N, Meli R, Autore G, Capasso F (1988b) Evidence against a dependence of the senna effect on prostaglandin formation. Pharmacology 36 (Suppl 1): 92-97

McCance RA, Widdowson WM (1955) Old thoughts and new work on bread white and brown. Lancet 2: 205-210

Mc Clure Browne JC, Edmunds V, Fairbairn JW, Reid DD (1957) Clinical and laboratory assessments of senna preparation. Br Med J 1: 436-439

McConnell AA, Eastwood MA, Mitchell WD (1974) Physical characteristics of vegetable foodstuffs that could influence bowel function. J Sci Food Agric 25: 1457-1464

Mc Naughton WK, Gall DG (1991) Mechanisms of platelet activating factor-induced electrolyte transport in the rat jejunum. Eur J Pharmacol 200: 17-23

Meisel JL, Bergman D, Graney D, Saunders DR, Rubin LE (1977) Human rectal mucosa: proctoscopic and morphological changes caused by laxatives. Gastroenterology 72: 1274-1279

Mereto E, Ghia M, Brambilla G (1996) Evaluation of the potential carcinogenic activity of senna and cascara glycosides for the rat colon. Cancer Lett 101: 79-83

Milner P, Belai A, Tomlinson A, Hoyle CV, Sarner S, Burnstock G (1992) Effect of long-term laxative treatment on neuropeptides in rat mesenteric vessels and caecum. J Pharm Pharmacol 44: 777-779

Moreto M, Gonalons E, Mylonakis N, Giraldes A, Torralba A (1979) 3,3-bis-(4-hydroxyphenyl)-7-methyl-2-indolinone (BHMI), the active metabolite of the laxative sulisatin. Arzneimittelforschung 29: 1561-1564

Moriarty KJ, Dawson AM (1984) Use and abuse of cathartics. In: Csaky TZ (ed) Pharmacology of intestinal permeation II. vol 70. Springer-Verlag, Berlin Heidelberg New York, pp 509-531

Moriarty KJ, Silk D (1988) Laxative abuse. Dig Dis Sci 6: 15-29

Mori H, Sugie S, Niwa K, Takahashi M, Kawai K (1985) Induction of intestinal tumors in rat by chrysazin. Br J Cancer 52: 781-783

Mori H, Sugie S, Niwa K, Yoshimi N, Tanaka T, Hirono I (1986) Carcinogenicity of chrysazin in large intestine and liver of mice. Jpn J Cancer Res 77: 871-876

Mori H, Yoshimi N, Iwata H, Mori Y, Hara A, Tanaka T, Kawai K (1990) Carcinogenicity in rats: induction of large bowel liver and stomach neoplasms. Carcinogenesis 11: 799-802

Muller SO, Eckert I, Lutz WK, Stopper H (1996) Genotoxicity of the laxative drug components emodin, aloe-emodin and danthron in mammalian cells: Topoisomerase II mediated? Mutat Res Genet Toxicol 371: 165-173

Muller-Lissner SA (1993) Adverse effects of laxatives: fact and fiction. Pharmacology 47: 138-145

Muller-Lissner SA (1993) Laxative-induced damage to the colon. In: Guslandi M, Braga PC (eds) Drug-induced injury to the digestive system. Springer-Verlag, Berlin Heidelberg New York, pp 131-142

Munch JC, Calesnick B (1960) Laxative studies. Human threshold doses of white and yellow phenolphthalein. Clin Pharmacol Ther 1: 311-315

Nakamura GJ, Schneiderman LJ, Klauber MR (1984) Colorectal cancer and bowel habits. Cancer 54: 1475-1477

Nell G, Rummell W (1984) Action mechanisms of secretagogue drugs. In: Csaky TZ (ed) Pharmacology of intestinal permeation II, vol 70. Springer-Verlag, Berlin Heidelberg New York, pp 461-508

Newal CA, Anderson LA, Phillipson JD (1996) Herbal Medicines. The Pharmaceutical Press, London

Nijs G, de Witte P, Lemli J (1991) Role of prostaglandin E2 in the secretion caused by rheinanthrone and rhein anthraquinone in the small intestine. Gastroenterology 100: A698

Nishioka I (1985) Discovery of new biological activities and the active components in rhubarb. In: Takemi T, Hasegava M, Kumagai A, Otsuga Y (eds) Herbal Medicine: kampo, past and present. Tsumura Juntendo Inc, Tokio, pp 41-51

Nusko G, Schneider B, Muller G, Kusche J, Hahn EG (1993) Retrospective study on laxative use and melanosis coli as risk factors for colorectal neoplasma. Pharmacology 47 (Suppl 1): 234-241

Odenthal K, Ziegler D (1988) In vitro effects of anthraquinones on rat intestine and uterus. Pharmacology 36 (Suppl 1): 57-65

Ornstain MH, McLain Baird I (1987) Dietary fiber and the colon. Mol Aspects Med 9: 41-67

Osten JR, Naterson BJ, Rogers AJ (1980) Laxative abuse syndrome. Am J Gastroenterol 74: 451-458

Painter NS, Almeida AZ, Colebourne KW (1972) Unprocessed bran in treatment of diverticular disease of the colon. Br Med J 1: 137-140

Parry E, Shields R, Turnbull AC (1970) Transit time in the small intestine in pregnancy. J Obstet Gynaecol Br Commow 77: 900-901

Parsons DS (1968) Methods for the investigations of intestinal absorption. In: Code CF (ed) Handbook of physiology, alimentary canal, vol III. American Physiological Society, pp 1177-1216

Passmore AP, Wilson-Davies K, Stoker C, Scott ME (1993) Chronic constipation in long stay elderly patients: a comparison of lactulose and senna-fiber combination. Br Med J 307: 769-771

Phillips SF, Gaginella TS (1977) Intestinal secretion as a mechanism in diarrheal disease.In: Jerzy-Glass GB (ed) Progress in gastroenterology, vol III. Grune and Stratton, New York, pp 481-504

Pinto A, Calignano A, Mascolo N, Autore G, Capasso F (1989) Castor oil increases intestinal formation of platelet activating factor and acid phosphatase release in the rat. Br J Pharmacol 96: 872-874

Powell DW (1983) Neurohumoral control of intestinal secretion. In: Turnberg LA (ed) Intestinal secretion. Knapp Drewett and Sons, Great Britain, pp 42-45

Prochnow L(1911) Experimentelle Beiträge zur Kenntnis der Wirkung von Volksabortiva. Arch Int Pharmacodyn 21: 313-319

Racagni G, Cantaluppi S, Fumagalli R (1986) Farmacologia generale ed applicata. Masson, Milano, p 749

Rachmilewitz D, Karmeli F, Okon E (1980) Effects of bisacodyl on cAMP and prostaglandin E2 contents, Na-K-ATPase, adenylylcyclase, and phosphodiesterase of rat intestine. Dig Dis Sci 25: 602-608

Rask-Madsen J, Bukhave K (1981) The role of prostaglandins in diarrhoea. Clin Res Rev 1 (Suppl 1): 33-48

Rask-Madsen J, Bukhave K (1983) Prostaglandins and intestinal secretion. In: Turnberg LA (ed) Intestinal secretion, Knapp Drewett and Sons, Oxford, pp 76-83

Rawson MD (1966) Cathartic colon. Lancet 1: 1121-1124

Refit (1996) Repertorio fitoterapico. OEMF, Milano

Riemann JF, Schenk J, Ehler R, Schmidt H, Koch H (1978) Ultrastructural changes of colonic mucosa in patients with chronic laxative misuse. Acta Hepato-Gastroenterol 25: 213-218

Riemann J, Schmidt H, Zimmerman W (1980) The fine structure of colonic submucosal nerves in patients with chronic laxative abuse. Scand J Gastroenterol 15: 761-768

Robbers JE, Speedie MK, Tyler VE (1996) Pharmacognosy and pharmacobiotechnology. Williams and Wilkins, Baltimore, p 51

Roggin GH, Banwell JG, Yardley JH, Hendrix TH (1972) Unimpaired response of rabbit jejunum to cholera toxin after selective damage in villus epithelium. Gastroenterology 63: 981

Roncucci L, Di Donato P, Carati L, Ferrari A, Perini M, Bertoni G, Bedogni G, Paris B, Svanoni F, Girola M (1993) Antioxidant vitamins or lactulose for the prevention of the recurrence of colorectal adenomas. Dig Colon Rectum 3: 227-234

Rondanelli R, Autelli F, Guaglio R (1980) Valutazione delle interazioni nelle associazioni tra farmaci. Bertolli A, Mascherpa P, Storti E (eds). ESAM, Roma

Rosprich G (1980) Dauerbehandlung mit Laxantien. Therapiewoche 30: 5836-5837

Rudolph RL, Mengs U (1988) Electron microscopical studies on rat intestine after long-term treatment with sennosides. Pharmacology 36 (Suppl 1): 188-193

Sarna K, Otterson M (1988) Gastrointestinal motility: some basic concepts. Pharmacology 36 (Suppl 1): 7-14

Sarner M (1976) Problems caused by laxatives. Practic 216: 661-664

Saunders DR, Sillery J, Rachmilewitz D (1975) Effect of dioctyl sodium sulpho-succinate on structure and function of rodent and human intestine. Gastroenterology 69: 380-386

Saunders DR, Sillery J, Rachmilewitz D, Rubin CE, Tytgat GN (1977) Effect of bisacodyl on the structure and function of rodent and human intestine. Gastroenterology 72: 849-856

Saunders DR, Sillery J, Surawica C, Tytgat GN (1978) Effect of phenolphthalein on the function and structure of iodent and human intestine. Dig Dis Sci 23: 909-913

Schmidt A, Von Noorden C (1936) Klinik der Darmkrankheiten, 2nd edn. Bergmann, Munich, p 382

Schultz SG, Zalusky R (1964) Ion transport in isolated rabbit ileum. I. Short-circuit current and Na+ fluxes. J Gen Physiol 47: 567-584

Schwartz WB, Relman AS (1953) Metabolic and renal studies in chronic potassium depletion resulting from overuse of laxatives. J Clin Invest 32: 258-271

Scott RS (1965) Management of constipation in obstetrics: A clinical report on 592 cases. West Med 6: 342-344

Shelton MG (1980) Standardized senna in the management of constipation in the puerperium. S Afr Med J 57: 78-80

Siegers CP (1992) Anthranoid laxatives and colorectal cancer. Trends Pharmacol Sci 13: 229-231

Siegers CP, von Hertzberg Lottin E, Otte M, Scheider B (1993) Anthranoid laxative abuse - a risk for colorectal cancer? Gut 34: 1099-1101

Smith B (1968) Effect of irritant purgatives on the myenteric plexus in man and the mouse. Gut 9: 139-143

Smith B (1973) Pathologic changes in the colon produced by anthraquinone purgatives. Dis Colon Rectum 16: 455-458

Smith CW, Evans PR (1961) Bowel motility. A problem in institutionalized geriatric care. Geriatrics 16: 189-192

Sonnenberg A, Muller AD (1993) Constipation and cathartics as risk factors of colorectal cancer: a meta-analysis. Pharmacology 47 (Suppl 1): 224-233

Speare GS (1951) Melanosis coli. Experimental observation on its production and elimination in twenty-three cases. Am J Surg 82: 631-637

Spiessens C (1991) Morphological and functional changes induced by laxatives in the intestinal mucosa. Thesis, Katholicke Universiteit, Leuven, p 145

Spiessens C, de Witte P, Geboes K, Lemli J (1991) Experimental induction of pseudomelanosis coli by anthranoid laxatives and non-anthranoid laxatives. Pharmaceut Pharmacol Lett 1: 3-6

Staumont G, Fioramonti J, Frexinas J, Bueno L (1988) Changes in colonic motility induced by sennosides in dogs: evidence of a prostaglandin mediation. Gut 29: 1180-1187

Steer HW, Colin-Jones DG (1975) Melanosis coli: studies on the toxic effects of irritant purgatives. J Pathol 115: 199-205

Stewart JJ, Gaginella TS, Bass P (1975a) Action of ricinoleic acid and structurally related fatty acids on the gastrointestinal tract. Effects on smooth muscle contractility in vitro. J Pharmacol Exp Ther 195: 347-354

Stewart JJ, Gaginella TS, Olsen WA, Bass P (1975b) Inhibitory actions of laxatives on motility and water and electrolyte transport in the gastrointestinal tract. J Pharmacol Exp Ther 192: 458-467

Sund RB, Lauterbach F (1986) Drug metabolism and metabolite transport in the small and large intestine: experiments with 1-naphthol and phenolphthalein by luminal and contraluminal administration in the isolated guinea pig mucosa. Acta Pharmacol Toxicol 58: 74-83

Sund RB, Lauterbach F (1987) 1-Naphthol metabolism and metabolite transport in the small and large intestine. Effects of sulphate and phosphate ion omission, and of 2,6-dichloro-4-nitrophenol in the isolated guinea pig mucosa. Pharmacol Toxicol 60: 262-268

Sund RB (1989) Pharmacokinetics of diphenolic laxatives. A status report. In: Koster AS, Richter E, Lauterbach F, Hartmann F (eds) Progress in pharmacology and clinical pharmacology, vol 7/2. Gustav Fischer Verlag, Stuttgart, pp 300-310

Tamai H, Gaginella TS (1993) Direct evidence for nitric oxide stimulation of electrolyte secretion in the rat colon. Free Radic Res Comm 19: 229-239

Thompson GW (1979) The irritable gut, functional disorders of the alimentary canal. University Park Press, Baltimore, p 275

Thompson WG (1980) Laxatives: Clinical pharmacology and rational use. Drugs 19: 49-58

Tidmarsh CJ (1936) Chronic indigestion. Longman's Green, Toronto, p 143

Tikkanen L, Matsushima T, Natoris S (1983) Mutagenicity of anthraquinones in the salmonella pre-incubation test. Mutat Res 116: 297-304

Tonini M, Costa M (1990) A pharmacological analysis of the neuronal circuitry involved in distension-evoked enteric excitatory reflex. Neuroscience 38: 787-795

Toyoda K, Nishikawa A, Furukawa F, Kawanishi T, Hayashi Y, Takahashi M (1994) Cell proliferation induced by laxatives and related compounds in the rat intestine. Cancer Lett 83: 43-49

Travell J (1954) Pharmacology of stimulant laxatives. Ann NY Acad Sci 58: 416-425

Turnberg LA, Bieberdort FA, Morawski SG, Fordtran JS (1970) Interrelationship of chloride bicarbonate, sodium and hydrogen transport in the lumen ileum. J Clin Invest 49: 557-561

Tyler VE, Brady LR, Robbers JE (1988) Pharmacognosy, 9th edn. Lea and Febinger, Philadelphia, pp 60-62

Tyler VE (1994) Herbs of choice. The therapeutic use of phytomedicinals. Pharmaceut Products Press, New York, pp 39-71

Tytgat GNJ, Mathus-Vliegen L (1983) Laxatives-laxative abuse-cathartic colon. J Drug Res 8: 1844-1850

Tzavella K, Schenkirsch S, Riepl RL, Odenthal KP, Leng-Peschlow (1995) Effect of long-term treatment with anthranoids and sodium picosulphate on the contents of vasoactive intestinal polypeptide, somatostatin and substance P in the rat colon. Eur J Gastroenterol Hepatol 7: 13-20

Ussing HH, Zehran K (1951) Active transport of sodium as the source of electric current in the short-circuit isolated from skin. Acta Physiol Scand 23: 110-127

Vago O (1969) Toxische und kaustische Komplikationen durch Gebrauch sogenannter fruchtabtreibender Arzneimittel. Z Geburtshilfe Gynakol 170: 272-277

Verhaeren E (1980) Mitochondrial uncoupling activity as a possible base for a laxative and antipsoriatic effect. Pharmacology 20 (Suppl 1): 43-49

Wager HP, Melosh WD (1958) The management of constipation in pregnancy. Q Rev Surg 15: 30-34

Wald A, van Thield DH, Hoechstaller L, Gavaler JS, Egler KM, Varm R, Scott L, Lester R (1982) Effect of pregnancy on gastrointestinal tract. Dig Dis Sci 27: 1015-1018

Wallace JL, Whittle BJR (1986) Profile of gastrointestinal damage induced by platelet-activating factor. Prostaglandins 32: 127-141

Wanitschke R (1980) Influence of rhein on electrolyte and water transfer in the isolated rat colonic mucosa. Pharmacology 20 (Suppl 1): 21-26

Wanitschke R (1987) Konsequenzen des Laxanzienabusus. Int Welt 5: 113-118

Weisbroadt NW (1987) Motility of the small intestine. In: Johnson LR (ed) Physiology of the gastrointestinal tract, 2nd edn. Raven Press, New York, pp 631-664

Werthmann MW, Krees SV (1973) Quantitative excretion of senokot in human breast milk. Med Ann Distr Columbia 42: 4-5

Westendorf J, Marquardt H, Poginsky B, Dominiak M, Shmidt J, Marquard H (1990) Genotoxicity of naturally occurring hydroxyanthraquinones. Mutat Res 340: 1-12

Wichtl M (1984) Teedrogen. Wisswnschaftliche Verlag-Gesellschaft, Stuttgart, pp 311-314

Wittoesch JH, Jackman RJ, Mc Donald JR (1958) Melanosis coli. General review and a study of 887 cases. Dis Colon Rectum 1: 172-180

Yagi T, Miyawaki Y, Nishikawa T, Yamauchi K, Kuwano S (1988) Involvement of prostaglandin E-like material in the purgative action of rheinanthrone, the intraluminal active metabolite of sennosides A and B in mice. J Pharm Pharmacol 40: 27-30

Yang K, Fan K, Mengs U, Lipkin M (1993) Effects of sennosides and non-anthranoid laxatives on cytochemistry of epithelial cells in rat colon. Pharmacology 47 (Suppl 1): 196-204

Subject Index

A

absorption, 2
acemannan, 29
acetylcholine (Ach), 16
aches, 55
acid
  alginic, 36, **39**
  cinnamic, 30
  citric, 42
  oleic, 35
  ricinoleic, 32
  salicylic, 30
acidosis, 4
adenomas, 53, 57, 58
adhesions, 44
adsorption, 61
aflatoxin, 59
agar, 36, 40
agents
  antiseptic, 30
  bulk-forming, 2
Agiolax®, 26, 39
aldosterone, 61
alkalosis, 56
alizarin, 59
alga, 39
algin, 39
allergic reaction, 39, 40, 48
aloe, 26, 29, 60
Aloe, 26, **29**, 60
  africana, 23, 29
  barbadensis, 23, 29
  Cape, 29
  Curacao, 29
  ferox, 23, 29
  gel, 29
  spicata, 29
  succotrina, 23
  vera, 23
aloe-emodin, 24, 27
aloe-emodinanthrone, 24
aloins, 24, 29

Althaea officinalis, 40
amphetamines, 8
anal
  abscesses, 4
  arctation, 4
  canal, 21
  fissure, 4
  sphincters, 21
anorexia, 4, 28
anthracene, 23
anthranoids, 3, 16, 25
anthraquinones, 4, **23**, 34, 42, 47, 51, 55, 57, 60
aperient, 3
apoptosis, 58
Arachis hypogaea, 35
L-arginine, 16
asthenia, 28
autacoids, 8, **15**, 19, 23

B

Bacteroides fragilis, 27
barbaloin, 29
betamannan, 29
benzodiazepines, 8
benzothiadiazide, 8
bile, 11, 32, 37
  acids, 3, 7, 37, 39
  salts, 14, 26
bisacodyl, 4, **49**, 55, 59
bismuth, 8
blackberries, 41
blood urea nitrogen, 31
boldo, 28
bradykinin, 15,18
bran, 4, **37**
brush border, 13

C

calcium, 34
  channel blockers, 8
  compounds, 8